In Praise of *TED* for Diabetes*

"*TED* for Diabetes* is a valuable story of personal discovery and empowerment. It is an excellent account of one person's road to self discovery.... . A *must read* for anyone dealing with the challenges of diabetes and the health care providers who impact them every day. The *TED** principals are simple tools that *power* empowerment!"

—**Donna Rice**, *President, Diabetes Health and Wellness Institute, Dallas, TX*

"In *TED* for Diabetes*, David Emerald and Dr. Conard have done an impressive job of offering a positive approach to managing not only diabetes, but any chronic medical challenge. Their vivid descriptions of the roller coaster of emotions, and relationship challenges, which accompany health issues, set the stage for the concise and clear introduction of tools for shifting attitudes and taking positive 'baby steps' to successful health management. Patients, their families, and their health care providers will all be grateful for this new perspective."

—**Ann V. Deaton**, *PhD, PCC, Leadership Coach and Clinical Health Psychologist*

"This book should be in the hands of all who seek individual responsibility for their health."

—**Wayne Andersen**, *M.D., author of Dr. A's Habits of Health, Medical Director of Medifast; and Co-Founder of Take Shape for Life*

"This incredible book can help change the lives of people with diabetes, and those who support them.

When a patient receives a diagnosis of diabetes, they often feel overwhelmed by all of the new medical and lifestyle information they receive. The authors provide real strategies for empowering people to better manage their own disease. I also think this book is a powerful and helpful tool for clinicians as it can educate and improve their ability to enable their patients to maintain a healthy lifestyle."

—**Dana McCormick**, *BS Pharm, RPh, Past President, American Diabetes Association, North Texas Chapter*

"David Emerald's 'The Empowerment Dynamic' (TED*) framework is one of the simplest, most powerful models I know of for optimal living. In *TED* for Diabetes*, David and Dr. Conard apply this framework to one of the greatest health challenges facing our world today--providing the inspiration and tools for everyone suffering from diabetes to shift and respond to the challenge as a Creator rather than as a Victim. If you'd like to optimize your health rather than just slow down the illness, this book is for you!"

—**Brian Johnson**, *Philosopher & CEO of en*theos Academy for Optimal Living; creator of PhilosophersNotes*

"*TED* for Diabetes* will take you on an inspiring and informative journey of discovery and hope. This compelling story is for anyone who is struggling with coming to terms with diabetes. It offers an entirely different window from which to view and approach diabetes. This book will put you firmly in the driver's seat. With a gentle approach and a dash of humor, authors David Emerald and Scott Canard, M.D., provide an easy to use recipe--complete with practical tools and the resources--for living the life you always wanted--even with diabetes. I highly recommend this book."

—**Donald Altman**, *M.A., LPC, author, Eat, Savor, Satisfy: 12-Weeks to Mindful Eating and One- minute Mindfulness*

"*TED* for Diabetes* takes the mystery out of empowering self and others. Personal empowerment is the missing active ingredient for optimal health, healthcare reform, the activated patient, the elimination of health disparities and the promotion of health literacy. If you want to get healthy, effectively support a person living with diabetes or just get a life, this transformative little book is the place to start."

—**Sandra Smith**, *PhD, MPH, Executive Director, Center for Health Literacy Promotion*

"This book is more effective than having a personal chef and health coach live with you, better than a month long yoga retreat in Bali, and yes, better than a magic pill to fix whatever ails you. Why? Because the *TED* framework changes you, from the inside, releasing the inner power you need to create optimal health. Reading this book will help you hold onto and express that power. That, my friend, is deep, true health."

—**Jennifer Louden**, *author of The Woman's Comfort Book and The Life Organizer*

TED*

FOR DIABETES

A Health Empowerment Story

Also by David Emerald

The Power of TED* (*The Empowerment Dynamic)

A Personal Guide to Applying The Power of TED* (*The Empowerment Dynamic)

Also by Scott Conard, M.D.

The Seven Healers

Weight Loss the Jabez Way

7 Keys to Adding Years to Your Life

The Seven Numbers

TED*

(*THE EMPOWERMENT DYNAMIC)

FOR DIABETES

A Health Empowerment Story

**David Emerald &
Scott Conard, M.D.**

POLARIS PUBLISHING
Bainbridge Island, Washington

TED*

(*The Empowerment Dynamic)
FOR DIABETES
A Health Empowerment Story

Printed in the United States of America

Published by Polaris Publishing
321 High School Road N.E., Suite D-3, PMB 295
Bainbridge Island, WA 98110

First Edition
Cover and Interior Design by JAAD
Cover Photo by Rick Braveheart

Library of Congress Cataloging-in-Publication
Data available
ISBN: 978-0-9771441-6-7

10 9 8 7 6 5 4 3 2 1
20 19 18 17 16 15 14 13 12 11

CONTENTS

DISCLAIMER

The information in this book is not intended or implied to be a substitute for professional medical advice, diagnosis or treatment or a substitute for professional psychiatric or psychotherapeutic evaluation or diagnosis. All content, including text, graphics, images and information, contained in this book is for general information purposes only. Polaris Publishing and its authors make no representations and assume no responsibility for the accuracy of information contained within the book and such information is subject to change without notice. Additionally, Polaris Publishing and its authors are not liable for any advice, course of treatment, diagnosis or any other information, services, or products available through the reading of this book or contained within the websites of Polaris Publishing or the authors.

FOREWORD

Every Day. As a mature single man with type 2 diabetes I think about what and when I will eat; how much insulin to inject; when to take my prescription medicine; when and how much to exercise (I am a runner); how much sleep to schedule; and how many hours I will work: every single day. "Exercising personal agency" is the phrase often used to describe a person who is actively managing a chronic disease. In other words, I am the agent responsible for my own health. As one doctor described it, "diabetes is the one major chronic illness in which the patient retains a degree of agency in terms of being well or sick, and it takes constant decision making and follow-through to accept and use that agency in a strong way." I am not a better person because of strong agency, but I am certainly a healthier person.

It all began for me on February 11, 1999. My Dad died that afternoon at the age of 77, and three hours later, at the age of 52, I was diagnosed with type 2 diabetes. My Dad also had diabetes, but I didn't know that until after his death. I learned this when my sister offered me his diabetes paraphernalia, which was too old to use, but it did wake me up about his condition.

I remember walking out of Dr. Rothman's Berkeley office in a daze that sunny Thursday afternoon after my diagnosis. Immediately, I switched into coping mode in order to fly home for my Dad's funeral, prepare and present a eulogy at the memorial service, and visit with my siblings and extended family. My memory of those events is sketchy because I was on autopilot and much of what was done and said hardly registered. I had to put diabetes out of my mind until I returned home; I felt I was on my own with this new reality. Since then I have realized that each of us with diabetes, even those surrounded by loving families and friends, are alone to an extent. As lonely as it can be, we must face ourselves and the magnitude of changes that come with this diagnosis.

I grew up in an alcoholic family where the universal rules of dysfunctional families were all operational: don't talk, don't trust, and don't feel. Following our Dad's example, my siblings and I didn't talk about his alcoholism or his diabetes. I wasn't surprised that I didn't know, but I was glad to find out that my diabetes didn't appear out of nowhere. There is a genetic link, although the medical profession readily admits that they don't know much about it. My assumption is that my Dad's alcoholism contributed to his adult onset diagnosis. I am not an alcoholic, but I am a workaholic and I am sure that my lifestyle contributed to my adult onset diagnosis. Very few adult children escape addiction in some form when they are raised in an addictive family system. And now it is clear that I had not avoided addictive tendencies or the family history of diabetes. But what was I going to do about it?

According to the Diabetes Research Institute (www.diabetesresearch.org) there are 4,110 new cases of diabetes diagnosed every single day. Was I typical? What did this mean? My doctor tried to explain what was going on, but much of what he said was not making an impact. My array of intense symptoms, though, was my biggest prod. I had all the classic symptoms, lingering fatigue, frequent urination, unquenchable thirst, increased hunger, and especially, blurred vision. As an editor in the book publishing industry, I earned my living by reading manuscripts and blurry vision was raising havoc in my life. My vision was blurred for eight straight weeks and my ability to read was greatly hampered. I worked hard to lessen my symptoms with little success and I was very frustrated. Type 2 diabetes doesn't happen all at once and getting "control" over it also doesn't happen quickly.

Fortunately, I was not as alone in my attempts to manage this new health issue as I had thought. One of my best friends at the time, the Rev. Tony Petrotta, said that he would go running with me every day and he would help me train to get in shape for races. This would give me a reason to run consistently, and it worked and still does. Another good friend, J. Walker Smith, who had type 1 diabetes, and was also a runner, said he would help me learn more about this disease and keep me on track by prodding me on a regular basis when I got lazy or complacent.

Frankly, I think these two men saved my life, even with my "exercising agency" inclination. I needed and wanted the support they offered and the impetus it provided for managing this chronic disease for the long haul. Both men were true to their word. I began the journey that every person with diabetes must embark on, whether he or she wants to or not: how to live daily with a chronic disease. Now, at least, I had help.

This book can be a great help to all who read it and take its guidance seriously. As people with diabetes, our biggest obstacles are not changing our diets, exercising, and taking medication. Our biggest challenge is finding a way to maintain the daily discipline of these required regimens, and changing our attitudes so that we don't get discouraged, frustrated, and lazy. This is the only book I know that confronts us with a new way of living that is more profound than just being told to "work harder!"

For ten of the last twelve years I have been able to manage my disease with diet, serious exercise, and medications. I had two relapses where my blood sugar levels flew through the roof because I got lazy about what I was eating. I was miserable and then had to work very hard to get back on track. Eventually my pancreas did not produce enough insulin and I had to start taking injections. I fought against taking insulin, as it seems everyone does since it is a controversial therapy, but Dr. Rothman, in his usual consistent and helpful manner, finally convinced me to try it. I don't know how rare it is, but I am most grateful to have a doctor who is friendly and firm with me. For more than a decade he has nudged me to try new things and be proactive about monitoring my health. He was right, of course, insulin turned out to be a wonderful gift that helped me stabilize my glucose levels. With his encouragement I learned how to integrate insulin injections into my daily routine. We all pray for a "cure" for diabetes but for me insulin is another life saver. As one of the more than forty million people in this country that doesn't have health insurance, I am also grateful that insulin is affordable for those of us on a very limited income.

At about the time I was switching to the use of insulin in my regimen, David Emerald came into my life and his first book, *The Power of TED** helped me become more aware of the psychological and emotional dimensions of dealing with any situation that made me feel sorry for myself. It contains language which reminds me of how important it is to "name" what is happening and, thereby, clarify what I can do about it. As with many who have this disease, I wanted it to suddenly disappear. I had many days when I felt victimized by it and by my family's health history. Fortunately, I was able to consult with David while he was writing a revised edition of his book and I became even more familiar with the language and concepts in his model and how helpful they are to readers.

Then another change happened: David was diagnosed with type 2 diabetes and our relationship now included a mutual area of concern. We provided some encouragement for each other and made sure we included this new topic in our conversations. David was also very motivated to exercise strong agency with his health and we understood each other's challenges and concerns more readily.

Through a series of connections and interactions, the idea for a book on Diabetes and the *Power of TED** began to emerge. David met Dr. Scott Conard, who is a medical expert in the field of diabetes care and management, and Scott was very interested in a collaborative effort to produce a book on this combined topic. Although I wasn't privy to their initial conversations, I could tell that this subject was percolating at a higher temperature for all of us.

What becomes quite clear to anyone who works with and gets to know David, and his wife Donna, is that they are talented, proactive, and creative people. Since they had learned a lot about writing and publishing with *The Power of TED**, it was not a great leap to do another book. They both bring many years of leadership and team building skills to any task: that was supremely the case with this book.

Within weeks of conversations *about* the project, we embarked on the project itself. Not surprisingly, the right people with the right skills, including Scott as a co-author, were quickly assembled into a team that could turn this idea into a book.

There are many books on diabetes. Over the years some of them have been helpful to me. In fact, you can search the shelves in a bookstore or scroll online through pages of book titles on most aspects of diabetes, primarily on the medical management, the nutritional guidelines, and the importance of diet and exercise. What I did not find were books that helped me understand the emotional, psychological, and spiritual dimensions of living with this disease. As someone who was personally and professionally curious about those aspects of life, I needed more than was available. David and Scott have addressed those issues in this book.

The team that wrote and produced the book you hold in your hands faced the challenge of writing a unique kind of book about this disease, and did so faithfully and with determination. The commitment and effort by the authors and the Polaris Publishing team to "get the word out" about diabetes have been herculean. Today it is estimated that twenty-six million people in the US have diabetes, including seven million who don't know it. I think it will be because of people like David and Scott and this book that hope can burn more brightly for those of us who live every single day with this disease. Maybe this book can help all of us become stronger agents for the management of our own health and turn this dreaded chronic disease into a gift that enriches our lives and the lives of those around us.

Roy M Carlisle
Alameda, California

INTRODUCTION

I am deeply committed to creating health empowerment. I see the occurrence of heart attacks, strokes, stages 3 and 4 cancer and diabetes as medical failures. In dealing with these diseases with each patient, we have a five to fifteen year window to prevent these conditions and to reverse their course - if not forever, then for years, possibly decades. I believe that we all do the best we can with the knowledge, training, and system in which we function, and the possibility of improving these variables is not only real, it is likely!

Over my years of practice, I have seen wonderful people struggle in their battle with prediabetes and diabetes. Many are lulled into the false security of the "I feel fine syndrome" when they don't understand the seriousness of their condition and its complications. Their efforts to manage diabetes are inconsistent, with periods of improvement followed by a loss of control, followed by a period of improvement, another loss of control, and so forth.

As a physician, I am frustrated and disheartened when I witness patients on an emotional roller-coaster with managing diabetes. While patients understandably feel victimized by the disease, I also know that there are choices they can make to live healthier and more fulfilling lives. Helping them see this possibility and take responsibility for managing their health is a challenge many in the medical profession face.

I changed my focus on illness as a physician when I was led to a small, easy-to-read book entitled *The Power of TED* (*The Empowerment Dynamic*) by David Emerald. The book was featured in the Stagen Leadership Institute's year long curriculum called "The Introduction to Leadership Program." Not only did we read it, but we examined how the shift from a "victim" mentality to a "creator" mentality opened the way to creating an empowered and engaged work place, transformed an organization's culture, and resulted in tremendous organizational success.

I met David when he was a guest faculty member for the Stagen Graduate Leadership Program the following year. After that session, we began to develop a close relationship sparked by the possibility of applying these principles to the medical patients served at my practice.

Applying the principles in the *Power of TED**
impacted all facets of my life, including my medical practice. In a significant job transition, I continued to practice the program outlined in the book
and found more and more success in my work and
in my family life. One of my responsibilities in the
new job was to help create the Medical Edge diabetes education program. As a part of this, we
attended the American Association of Clinical
Endocrinologists (AACE) National Meeting in
Seattle. I called David, who I knew lived in the
area, and was glad to hear that he was available
for lunch. While we ate, I noticed a change in his
demeanor and confidence as he shared that, after
switching doctors and going for his annual physical, he had just received some very distressing
news. Much to his surprise and disappointment,
seemingly from out of the blue, he had been diagnosed with type 2 diabetes.

It was then that our journey into this life transforming work for people with diabetes began.

With input from David, we began applying the
TED* insights and program to patients back at my
clinic. Soon we started seeing the shift that is taught
in this book; from the Dreaded Drama Triangle
(DDT), which you will learn about in the book, to
TED* as it led to breakthroughs in our patients'
health and wellbeing.

It was not unusual to see a person who had re-
cently been diagnosed with diabetes to reverse their

condition and no longer need shots or pills. To our delight, some individuals actually became an "un-diabetic" by shifting their mindset and taking daily "Baby Step" actions that created health, instead of just slowing their illness.

We then used these methods to address obesity, back pain, arthritis, and many other conditions. Soon these principles transformed people from the ups and downs of the DDT, to gradual improvement through applying TED* principles and practices, and eventually reaching and sustaining higher levels of health and wellbeing. Over weeks-to-years, Baby Steps became life transforming and the joy of watching patients experience success enriched both their lives and our own.

As I and my medical team gained more practice with the TED* principles, we saw demonstrable impact on our patients. I used every opportunity to nudge David into co-authoring a book on bringing *The Power of TED** to diabetes treatment and management.

It was during a lunch meeting with David and his wife, Donna Zajonc, that I shared the impact TED* was having in my life and in my practice. I once again asked David when we were going to write a book on TED* and diabetes. All of his previous responses to that question had been "Some day." This time he surprised me when he said "I am ready."

It takes time for a person to step into a resourceful and empowered relationship with a chronic disease. David was no exception. His personal journey while writing this book parallels the fictional character of the story: The ups and downs, the breakthroughs – all which lead to the character's pursuit of his life purpose, and his experience of health and well being.

It is in this spirit that David and I have written this book. If you have diabetes or another chronic condition, we hope that you too will experience the power that TED* delivers in life.

As you take your Baby Steps and see the flow of your life continually improve, we hope you will share your success with others and let us know the vitality and joy that you experience.

Committed to your success,
Scott Conard, M.D.
Dallas, Texas

CHAPTER

ONE

Out of the Blue

I was flabbergasted. All I managed to say was, "Wha...?"

The doctor looked at me over his reading glasses, "Joe, I am sorry to say that I think you have diabetes."

"How . . . how can that be?" I stammered.

"Let's look at the lab report here. See there?" he said, pointing to a printout with lots of numbers on it. "Your fasting blood glucose is over 200 and your hemoglobin A1c is 9.3. Not good," he stated.

"What does that mean?" I asked.

"It means that there is too much sugar in your bloodstream and your body is no longer dealing well with the sugar that it is taking in." He spoke solemnly and with a hint of exasperation, as if he had said this a thousand times.

"Simply put, either your body is resisting insulin or your pancreas is not producing enough insulin. When you eat refined sugar or starches like white bread, white rice, or processed pasta, your body converts all of these foods into sugar and your pancreas can no longer keep up.

"Insulin is a hormone created by the pancreas during the digestive process. It is also the key to moving the energy from the blood into the cells of the body. Without insulin, your cells don't get the energy they need.

"People with type 1 diabetes produce no insulin. But that is not your issue. Your situation is with type 2 diabetes.

"With type 2, during the early phase a person may produce over 10 times more insulin but the body's need for insulin still is not met. As the pancreas fails, the blood sugar gradually rises until insulin injections become necessary.

"Which treatment you need will vary depending on whether your body still produces enough insulin to meet its needs."

It was like he was speaking a foreign language to me. Pancreas? Insulin? Blood sugar? All I could do was stare back at him. I'm not sure I even blinked.

"Sorry to say, Joe, that unless you get on top of this, diabetes can cause additional serious consequences to your health. My hope is that we caught this soon enough to prevent – or at least significantly delay – these complications.

"I know it is a lot to take in all at once. We will give you some information that explains all this. I want you to have your blood drawn before you leave today. We need to double-check to confirm the diagnosis. I am pretty certain you have developed type 2 diabetes."

My mind was racing and I was about to ask the doctor how this could have happened when he looked down at his clipboard again, sighed slightly and said, "The last time you came for an exam was two years ago."

"It's been that long?" I asked as if I didn't know. It's easy putting off an annual exam. "I've been really busy with work and the kids and…"

The doctor looked carefully at the chart. "I see from your last few visits that your blood sugar has been creeping up. You've steadily put on weight too, haven't you?"

"Yes, I guess… a little." I looked down at the paunch that stretched my shirt out. I'm not that much heavier than I was three years ago, I thought to myself.

"My notes indicate that I told you to lose weight during both of those visits." Even though the doctor was about ten years younger than I was, I felt like a child being scolded. My head was spinning and I looked toward the door, wondering if I could escape from what I was hearing.

He continued, "How have you been sleeping lately?"

I said, "Now that you mention it, I'm tired a lot of the time – even during the day. I have to get up and pee a couple of times a night. Sometimes more. And it takes me a little while to get back to sleep. My wife complains because sometimes I wake her up too."

"Are you thirsty as well?"

"Yeah. I can't seem to drink enough these days. I carry a bottle of soda or a jug of iced tea around everywhere I go."

"Is that sweetened?"

I knew I was going to get dinged for my answer. "The diet stuff tastes awful to me. I mean, I try to, but…"

"Well, all that sugar is another contributor to developing diabetes. You have got to find an alternative."

He looked me in the eye and said sternly, "One more thing, Joe. When was the last time you had an eye exam?"

"It's strange that you ask," I replied. "It's been years, but I've noticed lately that I probably need a new prescription because things seem a little blurry. Eyesight fades with age, I guess."

He shook his head slightly. "Vision problems can also be a symptom of diabetes," the doctor said. He scratched his head. "You've got many of the classic symptoms, Joe."

Just then there was a light knock on the door. It opened and a nurse stuck her head in. "Sorry to interrupt. Doctor, the health insurance claims adjuster that you have been playing phone tag with is on the phone. You asked me to let you know."

The doctor looked at his watch and then at me. "Ask him to hold and I will be there in a couple of minutes."

My mind raced. "Why me? What have I done to deserve this?" The nurse closed the door and the doctor turned back to me.

"I don't get it." I protested. "I've never had any serious health challenges. I've never even spent a night in the hospital. How could I go from being normal to having diabetes?" I could feel the grip of fear in my gut.

The doctor said, "Joe, I don't mean to lecture, but this did not occur overnight, nor did it happen by accident. It takes time to develop diabetes. Sometimes there is a family genetic component, but not always. Regardless of your physical disposition, diabetes is usually brought on by the normal American lifestyle – things like an over-reliance on fast food and the lack of exercise. We all know there's an obesity epidemic, which is closely linked to the huge increase in diabetes.

"Unfortunately, you are one of the millions who are developing the disease. That is what is happening in America and other parts of the world these days." The doctor swung his arm in the air to demonstrate how widespread the epidemic had become.

He looked straight at me once again. "Your situation has been coming on for some time and I probably should have been more insistent in telling you to lose weight. But you've got no choice now. You have to change what you are eating and exercise more – bottom line. And I want you to start taking medication if your blood work confirms what I see here."

I stared at him, not knowing what to say in my defense. He quickly wrote out a prescription, tore it off, and handed it to me. I folded my arms like a little boy who was not going to eat his peas. "I don't want to take medication."

"Why not?"

"I haven't taken much more than a few aspirin over the years, except for antibiotics when I really needed them. I remember all the medications my parents seemed to be taking as they aged and I don't want to be like that."

"Have it your way for now, Joe." The doctor frowned. "But you have to face facts. From your glucose numbers and your symptoms, you have type 2 diabetes."

I just stared at him. "My nurse will be with you shortly." With that, he left the room. After softly tapping on the door, the nurse entered the room. She handed me a small stack of papers. She seemed rushed and said, "Here are some handouts with recipes, a list of possible complications, and ways to slow down the progression of the disease.

"Also, if you like, you can schedule an appointment with our dietician. The main thing, though, is to stay away from anything white – like bread, pasta, rice, donuts, and stuff like that. This sheet gives you some other diet tips, like reducing your intake of carbohydrates and fat."

I shook my head, "I expected to hear a lecture about my cholesterol, not diabetes. All I ever hear about is avoiding a heart attack. I feel blindsided."

She softened slightly and said, "A lot of people feel that way."

She then handed me a glucose meter. "This is yours to keep. Let me show you how to use it." She had me wash my hands and then pricked my finger with what she called a lancet. I flinched a bit. I've always hated needles. A little drop of blood emerged from my fingertip, which she had me place on a test strip that ran into the meter. After a few seconds the monitor beeped and gave a reading of my blood sugar. I didn't know exactly what the numbers meant, but I knew they weren't good.

She matter-of-factly ended by saying "There is an instruction book in here, along with a little journal for tracking your numbers. Follow these instructions very carefully.

"That's it for now. Don't forget to stop at the lab to have your blood drawn as you leave. Have a nice day."

Great, I thought to myself, more needles. With that, she was out the door. I obediently walked to the lab for a blood draw and then headed for my car.

As I opened the car door, the pile of pamphlets the nurse had given me slipped out of my hands and spread out on the pavement. *What is Diabetes?*, *Diabetes and Exercise*, *Know Your Diabetes ABCs*, *Managing Diabetes through Diet*. At least the glucose meter that the nurse gave me didn't fall to the ground. Even though I was shaken up, I really had no idea how much my life would change from this day forward.

Now What?

Driving home, the numbness was replaced by a flood of questions. What does this all mean? How will my family react? I actually thought about not telling them until I could figure things out. But I knew that I had to break the news to my wife, Lois, our 11th grade daughter, Lisa, and Joe Jr., our 9th grade son.

I thought about my weekly "burger nights" with Joe Jr. or JJ (as we call him). For years, he and I had been going to the diner and having a double cheeseburger, ketchup-drenched fries, and a large milkshake. "I guess those days are over," I actually said out loud.

And what about my friends? I was a regular on the bowling team. A bowling alley isn't the best place to find healthy food. Dinner on bowling nights was a Sloppy Joe, onion rings, and a beer or two.

The drive home was mostly on autopilot. I pulled into the driveway and into the carport. As I opened the door to the kitchen, I was first greeted by the seductive smell of something baking. Lois turned around from the oven and smiled.

HgbA1C (Hgb = hemoglobin) is a blood test that measures your average blood glucose level over the past 2 to 3 months. The A1C test is used to diagnose prediabetes and diabetes and is a helpful tool in tracking how well you are managing diabetes over time.

Blood glucose (also called blood sugar) is the main sugar found in the blood and the body's main source of energy. Contrary to popular myths, sugary food items don't "cause" diabetes. Keep in mind that most food is converted to glucose during the digestive process. Insulin, a hormone produced by the pancreas, then helps move this glucose into the cells to utilize the energy in the food we eat.

Fasting blood glucose test is a test used to diagnose prediabetes and diabetes, and to help people with diabetes track their illness. A "fasting" test means you haven't had anything to eat or drink for at least 8 hours, and provides your doctor with useful information about how your body is managing diabetes.

Diabetes is diagnosed if you have fasting blood glucose levels of 126 mg/dl or higher after not eating for over 8 hours on two separate occasions. If your fasting blood glucose levels are between 100 mg/dl (5.5 mmol/l) and 125 mg/dl (6.9 mmol/l), you have prediabetes and are at risk for developing type 2 diabetes and its complications.

HgbA1C to Average Daily Glucose Table (mg/dl and mmol/l) The average daily glucose means all of the blood sugars - before, during and after meals. Relating your short-term diabetes choices (daily diabetes care) to long-term diabetes choices (quarterly diabetes care results) can help you create baby steps to ongoing health. The higher the A1C and daily values, the more diabetes complications you are likely to experience.

AlC	eAG	
%	mg/dl	mmol/l
6	126	7.0
6.5	140	7.8
7	154	8.6
7.5	169	9.4
8	183	10.1
8.5	197	10.9
9	212	11.8
9.5	226	12.6
10	240	13.4

"Welcome home Sweetie! I made a cake for you to take to your monthly birthday lunch at work tomorrow and decided to make an extra one just for you," She said as she kissed me on the cheek. "Carrot cake with cream cheese icing – your favorite,"

I replied "That's too sweet."

"Thanks honey. I'm happy to do it."

"No," I said with a frown, "It's too sweet. I can't have it. I can't ever eat anything sweet again."

"What on earth are you talking about?"

"The doctor said I have diabetes," I announced, half expecting lightening to flash and thunder to roll.

Lois waved it off like a minor annoyance. "Oh, Joe," she said, "Don't be so dramatic. Certainly you can have one small slice." She passed the cake under my nose and smiled seductively.

Feeling guilty, I said, "You went to all that trouble, Lois. Hmm – it smells so good." I really felt torn because I knew it wasn't a smart thing to do, but I didn't want to disappoint my wife. "Well, maybe one small, very thin slice." I gave in. I was reaching for the cake when the news hit home for Lois.

"Are you serious? The doctor really said that you have diabetes?" She pulled the cake away from me. "Maybe you should wait until we find out more about this," she said.

"You're right. I don't know what I want or exactly what all I should do. I don't know how to deal with this idea of having diabetes." I plopped into a chair with a sad sigh, dumped the brochures and meter onto the table.

Lois put the cake down and sat down at the table with me. She picked up one of the brochures. "This talks about type 2 diabetes. Is that the kind you have?"

I nodded.

She asked, "There's more than one type?"

I said, "I... I guess so. I have no idea, really. No one explained that to me. They just said to me that I've got type 2."

"Maybe there is something the doctor can give you to cure it. Did the doctor give you medication for this?"

"No." I shook my head. "He wanted to, but I told him I didn't want to take anything. The doctor got a little annoyed with me when I wouldn't take the prescription."

She picked up another one of the brochures and read out loud, "'There's no known cure for diabetes.

Lifestyle changes are required for the remainder of life.' Oh, my!"

I read from a third brochure. "Diabetes can cause serious harm to the heart, kidneys, eyes, and nerves. It also is the leading cause of blindness and amputation in the U.S."

Tilting my head to the side I said sarcastically, "Great. I'm going to go blind and lose limbs over this thing!"

Lois crinkled her forehead like she does when she gets especially concerned and said, "I'm really getting worried about this now. Didn't you have an uncle with diabetes?"

"Oh, yeah. It was my dad's brother. I only saw him a couple times as a kid. I'd forgotten about that." I strained my brain to remember. "Lois, I just remembered that he had a fake leg. He used to tease me with it. I bet he had to have his foot amputated because of diabetes. I overheard my dad saying to my mom something about a blood disease taking his leg."

Lois's face grew more somber. "Look what it says in this pamphlet. They're selling identification bracelets so people will know you have diabetes." She leaned closer toward me. "Joe, this is really serious. I'm afraid it will change everything." I felt a dark blanket of despair fall over me.

Lois picked up the box with the glucose meter in it and asked, "What's this thing?"

"I'm supposed to use that several times every day – before and after every meal I think – to check my blood sugar." I explained. "I am supposed to prick my finger to test my blood. Can you believe this?"

She shook her head in disbelief. "Needles have never been your thing, Joe." Taking a deep breath and mustering determination to meet this head on, Lois said, "Well, let's try it out. Let's figure out how to use it."

As she read the directions, I told her the nurse had already demonstrated it and I pricked my finger. "Ouch! I hate this already!"

"This isn't going to be fun for anyone," she sighed.

That evening at dinner, we told the kids about my diagnosis. Before we got too far in explaining what we knew about diabetes, Lisa interrupted us. "I have been learning about diabetes in my health class when we were studying nutrition." She tossed her long brown hair back and forth the way she does when really excited. "We learned all about healthy eating. They even gave us a recipe book!"

Lisa paused, "Daddy, I don't mean that I am happy you have diabetes, but changing how we eat could be really cool! Some of my friends and I have been talking about becoming vegetarians. Maybe we could become a vegetarian family!"

"Give me a break!" JJ just rolled his eyes, crossed his arms and said, "No way am I giving up my burgers! Can't make a veggie out of me!"

Lois and I looked at each other in dismay. Already my health condition was launching us into a new level of family drama.

Giving It a Good Try

It took a few days – and the lab report I got in the mail from the doctor's office that confirmed the diagnosis – but I got over my initial shock and got down to business. I read all of the brochures I'd received at the doctor's office and went on the Internet to see what else I could learn.

There was a lot of information out there—mostly about diet, recipes and exercise--and I got a bit overwhelmed. However, I knew this was nothing to take lightly. I was really frightened by the serious impact diabetes could have on my long term health. The main points I saw over and over were:

* Type 1 diabetes is usually diagnosed in childhood when it is detected that the body does not produce insulin. Type 2, more commonly diagnosed in adults, occurs when your body either doesn't make enough insulin or ignores the insulin the body does make.

* Insulin is a hormone made by your pancreas that helps the glucose (a form of sugar), which is the result of digestion of food, move into the body's cells to produce energy.

* The symptoms of diabetes can be easy to overlook, as they may seem harmless, such as excessive thirst, frequent urination, fatigue and irritability.

* Diabetes can contribute to a number of medical problems. Because high blood sugar over-taxes

certain organs in the body – especially blood vessels, nerves and kidneys – it can lead to heart disease, kidney failure, non-traumatic lower limb amputation, stroke, and blindness.

And the statistics were shocking. I couldn't believe the millions of people around the world who had either prediabetes or type 1 or type 2 diabetes, and how rapidly the growth had occurred and how much it is accelerating. This was especially true in more developed countries.

Current Statistics

* 8.3% of the U.S. population has diabetes (25.8 million children and adults), of which about 7 million are undiagnosed (people have it, but don't yet know it)

* 7.1% of non-Hispanic whites have diabetes

* 8.4% of Asian Americans have diabetes

* 12.6% of non-Hispanic blacks have diabetes

* 11.8% of Hispanics have diabetes

* Type 2 diabetes is the most common form of diabetes (95% of people with diabetes). Other forms of diabetes include type 1 (insulin dependent), gestational and prediabetes.

* An estimated 79 million people in the U.S. have prediabetes (not officially diagnosed, but at increased risk of developing type 2 diabetes).

* Worldwide, the International Diabetes Federation estimates there are 246 million adults with diabetes.

It was pretty sobering stuff. The message was clear: lifestyle changes are the most effective way to prevent or delay type 2 diabetes complications. I had to lose weight. I had to change what I ate. I had to exercise more. I had to monitor my blood sugar levels several times a day.

I found and printed some diabetes meal plans in addition to the ones the nurse had provided, I gave them to Lois. She cooked different meals for Lisa and me than she did for herself and JJ. It was hard for me to eat new dishes and smaller portions, even with Lisa's enthusiasm, while watching Lois and JJ eat the food I loved.

I also started walking every other night. I'd never exercised much and was in front of a computer most of the day at work. But I was determined to get on top of my diabetes. At least I could do something and I was proud of myself for this significant effort.

Even though I hated pricking my finger, I checked my numbers just like I was instructed and plotted them in the booklet that came with my blood glucose meter. I waited eagerly for my efforts to show themselves in my numbers. But after about three weeks of making these sacrifices, not much changed. I still dragged through the day.

I tried switching to diet or unsweetened drinks, but I was thirsty and drank a lot, which meant I had to go to the bathroom at night.

In spite of my best efforts, my sugar level stayed about the same. I complained to Lois one afternoon,

"Nothing seems to be changing and I'm doing my best."

She patted me on the shoulder. "Haven't your numbers changed at all?" she asked.

"Not much," I said as I shook my head. In that moment I decided that it was useless to check my readings every day. "What's the point? All I get is bad news."

I decided that checking my blood sugar levels three times a week would be enough for me. With no reward for my effort, it got harder to keep up the walking, so I tried to get in at least two walks a week, mostly on the weekends. And, I'll admit, I snuck a piece of pizza from my daughter's birthday party. Before long, I was pretty much back to my old habits.

One afternoon, Lois reminded me, "Joe, your appointment with the doctor is next week."

"Thanks for reminding me," I said sarcastically. "I can't believe it has been nearly three months already."

"Yes, honey. How's your blood sugar been running in the morning?"

I said sheepishly, "The last time I took it, it was better." I didn't want to tell her my numbers were still well above the healthy range. "When was the last time you took it?" she asked.

I answered, "A couple mornings ago."

She frowned at me. "A couple of days ago? Aren't you supposed to do it several times a day?"

It was disheartening. I knew I'd better get my act together quickly if I was going to have a good score by my appointment. I went on the Internet to find a quick way to get my sugar level down, but everything I found was about exercise and eating right. Blah, Blah, Blah.

In my search, I stumbled upon a support group that met the following night at a hospital nearby. I'm not one for groups, but I figured someone there could tell me how to avoid being scolded by my doctor.

The next night I walked into the hospital and was directed downstairs to a conference room. It was what you'd expect—a room with folding chairs set in a circle with a whiteboard and a nurse named Andi as the leader. I took a seat and waited to see what would happen.

Andi gave a short talk on the importance of exercise and then opened it up for discussion. One group member after another complained about how hard it was to stay on their diets; how little time they had to exercise; and how little their efforts made on lowering their blood sugar levels. Andi responded with the same litany of explanations and warnings I had been reading about on the Internet. What I heard in the group matched what I had been experiencing. It seemed that no one there knew any more than I did, and I was just starting out!

I left very discouraged. I felt like I was alone in dealing with this disaster called diabetes.

Type 1 diabetes means your pancreas produces little or no insulin and you need daily insulin doses (via injection or pump) to survive. Type 1 diabetes develops most often in younger people and is not, at this time, preventable.

Type 2 diabetes is a disruption in your body's ability to convert the food you eat into energy.

People with type 2 diabetes can no longer properly use insulin, a hormone released by the pancreas during the digestive process. Type 2 diabetes tends to run in families (is genetic) but development of it is very much dependent on environmental factors (unhealthy diet and lack of exercise). The disease and its complications can be prevented and/or delayed with lifestyle changes (healthy habits that include eating well and consistent physical activity) as well as medication (pills and, eventually, insulin). Type 2 is the most common form of diabetes (95% of the diabetes population).

CHAPTER

TWO

Not Alone In the Drama

"Joe, I'm not at all happy about your numbers," the doctor said while studying my chart. "Your fasting blood glucose and A1c are still much too high."

I defended myself, "Well, that's better than before!"

He responded sternly. "Barely. It has been 3 months and you are down 17 on fasting blood sugar and a mere .5 on A1c. Your weight's not much better either. Have you been exercising and eating right?"

"I've tried," I said sheepishly. I hated being grilled like this.

"Well, numbers don't lie, Joe." He said firmly. "You're not taking this very seriously."

"I am too!" I protested. "I've been walking and my wife cooks me recipes I got off the Internet. I even went to a support group."

The doctor frowned at me. "Then I strongly urge you to go on medication."

It was my turn to look stern. "I don't want to do that, doctor. I don't like taking drugs."

He shook his head at me then turned back to the clip board as he wrote out a prescription. Tearing it off, he said, "Here, Joe. You really need to take this medication. Otherwise, you could suffer very serious complications."

I sat glaring at him, unwilling to take the paper. "I am not ready to go on meds." I stood up, "I'll find another way."

The doctor squared off with me and said "Look Joe, you have diabetes – there is no way around it. The sooner you accept this reality and start to take your medication, the better you will do. The medication will help you." I took the prescription slip, but had no intention of taking it to a drug store.

I fumed while heading out to the waiting room. I muttered to myself, "Why is he making it so hard on me? My levels were lower. That's improvement. He's not being fair about this." I glanced up at a display of fliers and one caught my eye. It read, "Are You Challenged by the Rollercoaster Ride of Managing your Diabetes?" I thought, man, am I ever! I picked it up and started reading while I walked to my car:

> You are not alone. Come experience a different kind of diabetes class and learn how to take a more empowered and resourceful approach to living with this chronic disease. *Empowered Living with Diabetes* is a six

session series that takes place on the 1st & 3rd Monday evenings of each month from 7 – 8 PM. Location: Edgecliff Community Center (2 blocks off Metro bus route 72).

I relaxed a bit and said to myself, this isn't working for me and I am not connecting with the doctor here at all. I know where I'm going to be next Monday night. Maybe there *is* a way out of this misery.

Over the next couple of days I did my best to keep my hopes up. Still, I moved through my days with a sense of dread. I felt all the more alone the following Monday evening when Lois and I were washing the dinner dishes. She asked me, "Isn't that diabetes meeting tonight?"

"Yeah, but I'm so tired. I didn't sleep well last night."

She cocked her head at me the way she does when she's annoyed. "Honey, how was your glucose level when you took it a few minutes ago?"

"It's up again." I tried to brush it off. "Sometimes it's up. Sometimes it's down."

"I don't want to preach at you, honey. But you didn't walk last night because of the rain, and I saw you sneak a few bites of ice cream after dinner tonight."

"You sound like the doctor." I was steamed. "I need support, not criticism. I told you, I'm too tired to go out tonight!" Just then the phone rang. It was Rob.

"Hey, buddy!" Rob said, sounding like he was underwater. "I've come down with a really bad cold. Can you sub for me tonight at the bowling league?"

"Sure, I can bowl for you." I replied quickly.

Lois said, "Oh, I thought you were too tired to go out."

I sighed. There was no arguing with Lois when she was in this sort of mood. "Well, actually Rob, I can't sub tonight. Lois just reminded me that I need to go to a class on diabetes." I bit my lip. I hadn't meant to tell any of my friends yet.

Rob gasped, "You have diabetes? When did that happen?"

"I just found out a couple of months ago. I'm handling it okay, but don't tell any of the other guys, okay? It's no big deal really."

Rob assured me, "Okay, man, but I feel for you. I have an aunt who is in a nursing home because of diabetes. Your secret is safe with me."

I must admit I felt pretty embarrassed, like I had a deep, dark secret. After Rob said he was sorry to hear about the diabetes, I hung up. Without looking at Lois, I grabbed my jacket. First the doctor and now Lois. I was being persecuted from all sides, it seemed.

As I drove to the community center, I felt really depressed about being diagnosed with diabetes. For the first time in a long while, tears actually started to well up. I was really scared and felt alone. The so-called support I was getting from Lois made me feel all the more isolated. No one understood what I was going through.

My New Friend SARAH

I didn't expect this group to be any different from my first experience, so my expectations were pretty low. I was relieved to see that the class was held in the lounge of the community center with a mixture of couches, stuffed chairs, and a few padded folding chairs. I thought to myself, this beats those hard chairs at the other group meeting.

Looking around the room, I was struck by the diversity of the group. It was a mix of ethnicities: Caucasian, African American, Latino, Asian, and someone who appeared to be a Native American. The age range, on the other hand, was not quite as diverse. There seemed to be a lot of people from my age group, meaning a lot of "baby boomers" in their 50s and 60s, with a few in their 40s. There were only a couple of younger people.

In spite of the more welcoming seating, many of people looked as uncomfortable as I felt. I sat down next to an older gentleman who smiled slightly. He introduced himself, "Hello, I'm Ram." He spoke with a slight Indian accent. His broad smile calmed me down a bit.

I greeted him and we both turned our attention to an attractive woman who appeared to be in her forties and who had just stood up in the front of the room. Her black hair was pulled back into a ponytail giving her a stylish, yet comfortable, look. She glanced around the room flashing a warm smile and said, "Welcome to all of you here tonight. My name is Marianne. I'm a nurse and Certified Diabetes Educator. I am also a person with diabetes. I was first diagnosed about 15 years ago."

She handed a stack of stapled papers to a class member near her and explained, "Please take one of the handouts that describes our six-session curriculum. Tonight is the first of the series, so that's fortunate for those of you who are here for the first time. But you can invite others to join in any time, as this is a rotating class. As soon as we finish the last class, the next week we start the sequence over again."

I took the handout packet, passed the rest on, and flipped through the pages. I was impressed with the thoroughness of her class write up. At least it appears she knows her stuff, I thought to myself.

Marianne said, "Before we begin, I want to be clear about one primary ground rule. Confidentiality is critical. For this class to be at its best, everyone needs to feel safe to share their experiences and to ask questions. So, what gets shared here stays here. Do we all agree?"

Heads around the room nodded in affirmation.

"Great! My first question is how many of you have been personally diagnosed with type 1 diabetes or have family members who have been diagnosed?" A few hands went up. "I'll assume the rest of you have a type 2 diagnosis, or you are here with or for a family member who does. The attendance in this class reflects the norm in the U.S. About 90 to 95% of those diagnosed with diabetes have type 2. A lot of my examples and focus will be about type 2, because that has been my personal experience. But I don't want those of you with type 1 is to feel left out. I am delighted that both are represented here. This class series speaks to all of our experiences.

"The topics we will cover are not about particular treatment protocols and modalities. It is about how you think and relate to your diabetes and, for that matter, to the whole of your life."

Calling our attention back to the packet, she gave an overview of the series. "Tonight we will begin by looking at how most people feel and react when we first receive a diagnosis of diabetes, and the drama it tends to create in our lives. In our next class, we will explore how our reactions to diabetes can keep us locked into what we call the 'roller coaster' pattern we often take in dealing with diabetes.

"In our third meeting, we will introduce you to a new and different mind-set from which to more effectively meet the challenges that diabetes presents. We will build on that mind-set in week four with a more resourceful and empowering way to relate to your diabetes, the healthcare professionals with whom you work, and your family and friends, for that matter.

"Week five will focus on a way of thinking and planning for how to live in an empowered way with your diabetes. In the final class, we will bring it all together through a simple process for taking day-to-day steps in creating health and wellbeing in your life – even in the face of diabetes."

She then asked if there were any questions about the logistics or the outline. The only one of substance was what one should do if they missed a class in the sequence. Her advice was to come to the next class and then to pick up the missed session during the next cycle.

"Ready to begin?" she asked. I nervously nodded in response.

"Let's start with your relationship to your diabetes and the kind of experience you have most likely had that led you to attend tonight."

She continued, "In this first class, I want to introduce you to SARAH. 'She' is not a person, but my guess is that you have met her through your process of coming to grips with your diabetes diagnosis. This is a typical cycle of emotions and reactions that we all go through when we learn we have diabetes." Marianne turned to the whiteboard and wrote in all capital letters:

S

A

R

A

H

Turning to the group, she said, "I'd like to hear how some of you found out you had diabetes. Who is willing to share?"

After a few minutes of awkward silence, a man finally raised his hand and said, "I had a heart attack. Even though I had sky high cholesterol, they said the heart attack was actually a result of my diabetes. I had no idea heart attacks were more common with diabetes."

Marianne nodded. "I think that's a common misconception among us. Diabetes and heart disease are often closely linked. Anyone else want to share?"

A woman on one of the couches spoke up. "I went to see my doctor because my feet went numb. He told me it was nerve damage from diabetes." She choked up a bit. "He says that the damage is permanent and now I walk with this," she pointed to her cane. "I'm in my late 50's and I already have trouble getting around."

Marianne explained to the class, "Nearly half of us with diabetes will suffer some kind of nerve damage. Sometimes the damage is temporary, but sometimes not." Marianne turned back to the woman, "I am so sorry to hear about your situation. I am committed to this class making a difference in how you deal with your situation. That is my intention for all of you here."

Right next to the woman on the couch was a younger man who offered, "I've worn glasses since I was in my teens. I'm used to getting new glasses every few years, so I didn't think much about it when my vision got a little blurry. I thought I just needed new glasses. But after my eye doctor ran some tests, he suggested I go see my family doctor, who confirmed his suspicion that my vision problems were diabetes related. I was stunned."

Marianne nodded, "Vision issues are also linked with diabetes. In fact, here's another statistic: 40 to 45% of Americans with diabetes have some level of diabetic vision issues. And we're twice as likely to get glaucoma as those without diabetes."

I leaned over the Ram, "Well, this is uplifting."

He smiled slightly and nodded.

As if hearing my comment, Marianne said, "But these statistics can be changed. And that's what we're here to talk about. I want all of you to think back to when you were first told you had diabetes. How many of you were shocked or, at least, surprised?" Nearly all the hands in the room went up. She wrote next to the S on the whiteboard: *Shocked/ Surprised*.

Ram raised his hand and added, "It also seems that *Sadness* could work there too." I nodded, thinking about how I had felt in the car driving to the class.

"That is a great point. Many people feel sad about the changes they face. I guess some good news is that shock, surprise, and even sadness don't typically last too long. They are usually followed by feelings and expressions of *Anger*," and she wrote "Anger" next to the A. "Is anyone willing to share how anger showed up for you?"

Again, silence greeted the question. Ram finally raised his hand and said with a self-effacing smile, "I got angry at my genes! Diabetes has run in my family for at least two generations – probably more."

A woman across the circle offered, "I was angry at my heritage, too…as if that could be changed…" She added, "But I was even more angry with my doctor for telling me. I am still furious that he doesn't have easy answers for me or some magic… something that would make it go away. Turns out all he does is criticize me and wants to give me more medication."

Then a realization struck me and I raised my hand. "You know," I stammered, "I've also been disturbed by my doctor for not being clear with me in the past that my diabetes has been coming on for some time. I'm also angry at myself. I should have listened to him and taken better care of myself."

Marianne said, "I know it is not easy. Anger comes and goes. What usually happens next is that anger gets replaced by *Rationalization*," which she wrote next to the R. "We find ways of denying, mini-mizing or hoping that diabetes will just go away."

No kidding, I thought.

"The good news," she said, "is that we can all move to the stage of *Acceptance*," which she added to the whiteboard next to the second A.

"Acceptance that you have a medical condition that needs to be – and can be – managed. You have come to this class and will, hopefully, attend the en-tire series of classes because now you are ready for help – and a good dose of hope." Next to the H, she wrote the words *Help* and *Hope*."

Hope, I thought to myself, Now, that's something I've not felt lately.

Marianne turned to the group and said, "Hope may sound a little strange to you at this point, but I can tell you this: if you stay with us and complete the full curriculum of this class, you will leave feeling more empowered and resourceful. Over time, as you grow in your understanding of the way to deal with diabetes, the fear, anxiety, and other negative emotions you are probably feeling will begin to dissipate.

"One of the biggest barriers we face in managing our diabetes and living fulfilling lives is the emotional barrier we face as we move from Shock into Anger, find our way through Rationalization, come to the point of Acceptance, and then reach out for Help and Hope."

She pointed back to the whiteboard as she said, "These are the stages we all go through when first dealing with the diagnosis of diabetes.

Shock/Surprise/Sadness
Anger
Rationalization
Acceptance
Help & Hope

"I know these stages myself because I went through them when I received my diagnosis. I was a single mother with a teenage daughter. I won't minimize the challenges and changes we faced. But we made it through. My daughter is now a well-adjusted adult who lives a healthy lifestyle because of what we learned together. And I am managing my diabetes well and am getting to do the work I love, which is helping you move through SARAH and to change the way you relate to your diabetes."

The Dreaded Drama Triangle (DDT)

Marianne explained, "In the first few classes, I need to ask for your patience because I know you want to jump right to the help and hope phase of SARAH. You can trust me when I say that we will eventually get to the place of health empowerment in a few more classes. But, first we must confront and understand how you are currently relating to your diabetes.

"The chances are very, very high that you are currently relating to your diabetes through the lens of the Karpman Drama Triangle, which we call the Dreaded Drama Triangle[1], or DDT," she said, emphasizing the three words as if they described a scary monster. A few people chuckled nervously.

Marianne drew a large, downward pointed triangle and wrote above it:

---

1   The Dreaded Drama Triangle (DDT) is based on the Karpman Drama Triangle, originated by Stephen B. Karpman, M.D (www.KarpmanDramaTriangle.com).

Dreaded Drama Triangle (DDT)

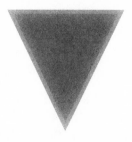

She said, "And no, it's not about the pesticide – though it is quite toxic in nature. When I was first diagnosed, I felt victimized," she told us. "I hated having to pay attention to what I ate, having to exercise and feeling different from everyone else around me. Why did they get to eat whatever they wanted? Why didn't they have to exercise every day? I was really unhappy. How many of you feel like you've gotten a rotten deal?" Most people held up their hands. I think mine was the first in the air.

She wrote Victim at the bottom of the triangle and said, "I suspect that most of you are feeling victimized, just like I did. None of us 'deserves' to have this disease.

"When we feel like something unfair has happened to us, we feel victimized. We take on the role of Victim when some important dream or desire that we care about has been denied or thwarted. When we receive the diagnosis of diabetes, the 'dream' of living our lives the way we always have is no longer available to us. We lament and say 'poor me' or 'why me?' or 'it's not my fault' – all forms of self-talk that a Victim engages in."

She nailed it for me again. I could feel the sadness in the pit of my stomach.

"There's an important distinction that I need to make here," Marianne turned to face us. Scanning the room she said with bright eyes and a slight smile, "While the reality is that you have been victimized by acquiring the disease, it does not mean you have to live in the state of Victimhood. There is a huge difference between Victimization and Victimhood." She wrote the two words on the board.

"Victimization happens to everyone at some level or another. It is situational. If, on a warm summer night someone yells in the street and awakens you, you are victimized as your desire for a good night's sleep is interrupted. Victimhood, on the other hand, is a label of we put on ourselves. Victimhood becomes a way of life, and colors all of our life experiences. It can even become our identity."

She explained, "The core purpose of this class series is to support you in responding, in an empowered way, to the victimization you are currently experiencing with your diabetes, while challenging you to not adopt a life stance of victimhood."

Marianne's words struck home. Until I'd heard the doctor say I had diabetes, I would never have considered myself a Victim. Yet, as she talked, I realized that I had definitely fallen into victimhood over the state of my health.

She continued, "In order to be a Victim, one must have a Persecutor," she said, as she wrote the word at the upper right point of the triangle.

Persecutor

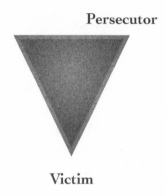

Victim

"A Persecutor can be a person. It can be a circumstance, like a natural disaster. Most relevant here is that it can be a condition, like diabetes. Regardless of whether it is a person, condition or circumstance, the Persecutor dominates the time and attention of the Victim."

She asked, "How many of you perceive the Persecutor of diabetes as dominating your life right now?" 100 percent of the hands shot up.

"Right," she replied, "and when we experience victimization by a Persecutor like diabetes, we feel powerless and dominated by it because of the dream or desire of a normal life is being taken from us."

Powerless and dominated is right, I said to myself and leaned forward in my chair as I wondered what the third point of the triangle would be.

"The Victim," Marianne explained, "feels power-less to cope with the Persecutor and turns to the third role in this drama. That role is the Rescuer." Marianne wrote Rescuer on the upper left corner of the triangle. "The Rescuer is most often a person, but it can also be anything that helps a Victim dis-tance themselves or numb out from their feelings of powerlessness, like drugs or alcohol or even com-fort food.

"We hope that a Rescuer is going to emerge and release us from the drama." She paused a mo-ment, and then asked, "Who or what have you been hoping would be your Rescuer?"

A woman in the front of the class nearly shouted, "My doctor! He was supposed to have all the an-swers, or a pill or something that would make it all better."

Marianne responded by looking around the room at others who were nodding in agreement with the statement the woman had made. "It also sounds to me that you expected your doctors to either protect you or save you from diabetes." Murmurs could be heard around the room.

Another woman in the back said with heavy sar-casm, "Well, they are called health care providers. Why don't they provide us with health care instead of waiting and then wanting to give us 'illness' care?"

"At the risk of sounding a bit defensive of my profession here," Marianne countered, "many health care professionals are firmly caught up in the drama themselves. I understand how anger can be directed at doctors or, I dare say, diabetes educators like myself, when we are not able to just fix it and make it go away. No one wants to be the one to deliver the harsh reality of the diagnosis or have to inform a patient about the changes that must be made to manage his or her life."

The group was quiet as we all took that in. I asked, "Do the doctors feel victimized by us?" I didn't like the sound of that.

Marianne smiled, "I suspect that many in the health care profession have simply given up trying to educate patients on self-care. How many times have your doctors told you to lose weight? Probably many times, but it's easy to brush off sound medical advice. The health professionals who are also caught up in the DDT feel powerless to help and so it is easy to stop trying to convince patients to change their ways."

Ram smiled, "Are you saying that health professionals are people too?" The group laughed.

Marianne joined in the laughter, "Yes, as unbelievable as that might seem at the moment, we're all human beings dealing with complex and difficult issues.

"The drama of diabetes, my friends, is bound up in the Dreaded Drama Triangle and the toxic interplay of the roles of Victim, Persecutor, and Rescuer," she concluded as she called our attention to a handout that had the completed diagram.

The Dreaded Drama Triangle (DDT)

Rescuer   Persecutor

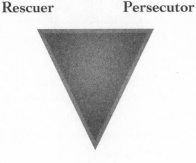

Victim

Marianne said, "Once engaged in the triangle, we tend to play all three roles and can see ourselves moving between them."

"What do you mean?" asked a middle-aged, balding man who had not spoken before.

Marianne responded, "When you feel or project anger toward your doctor, in which role are you seeing him or her at that moment?"

He thought for a minute, looked at the DDT diagram and said, "I guess I would be reacting to the doctor as a Persecutor who is not giving me an easy way out of my dilemma."

"Right!" Marianne declared, "And if you expressed your anger in some way towards your doctor, how do you think he or she would feel? What role would they be in?"

I thought about how my doctor had walked out of the exam room when I refused his advice to take medication. I raised my hand and confessed, "While

I felt like he was persecuting me," I paused and then added, "he probably felt like I was persecuting him."

"Probably so," Marianne agreed. "When our doctors don't meet our unrealistic expectations, we can view them as Persecutors."

Marianne continued, "So we can see how the DDT and all of its toxic dynamics make up the way we relate to our health challenge and the medical system. It's not a fun, nor very effective, way to live, is it? We can feel trapped.

"Let me be really personal here. The reason I developed this class series is because I felt victimized and trapped by my situation until I discovered a completely different way of relating to diabetes. I can't wait to share that with you, but it will be in a few more weeks, as I said."

I grunted. I wanted to know the answer now! But I paused for a moment, looking back over the past few days. I definitely felt like a Victim in this scenario. And, judging from the sad look I saw in Lois's eyes at times, she felt like a Victim too. That meant that she saw me as part of the problem— more like a Persecutor. Hmm...

My thoughts were interrupted by a lady down the row from me who said, "Marianne, to be honest, I see myself in all three roles. But now, we're waiting for the solution. You are going to tell us a way out of DDT, aren't you?"

It seemed like the group leaned forward together in anticipation of her answer.

Marianne smiled, "Don't look to me to be your Rescuer!"

The group groaned, understanding what she meant. We were all still caught up in the DDT dynamic. We wanted someone to save us from our victimization. However, I was disappointed by her response. I thought, I'll bet that at the end of this course, I'll be right where I started. If Marianne doesn't know the secret to overcoming diabetes, then I don't know where else to turn.

As if reading my mind, Marianne continued, "Don't lose heart. You will find hope and new ways of meeting the challenge of diabetes through this course."

On that encouraging note, Marianne dismissed us. Ram and I picked up our jackets and headed for the parking lot.

"That actually went by fairly quickly," I said to Ram.

Ram agreed. He said, "I feel like she described me perfectly, so hopefully she'll have more positive information in the next class."

I nodded. Ram asked, "Will I see you at the next class?"

"Yes, I'll be back." I left with an odd mixture of both hopefulness and apprehension. Sure, I'd found a resource and group of people that I felt I could learn with, but I still felt anxious. I guess that's why it is called the *dreaded* drama triangle. Marianne had so named my experience and the seeming merry-go-round of the past few months.

Remembering the flyer that had drawn me to the class, I thought, or maybe it is the roller coaster.

CHAPTER

THREE

Riding the Roller Coaster
with Diabetes

The sense of camaraderie I felt after Marianne's Monday class all but faded by Tuesday morning when I woke up and realized that I still had diabetes. I hadn't slept well and I dragged myself to the kitchen for a cup of coffee. My family was already eating breakfast, but I wasn't in the mood for small talk. I saw Lois wink at the kids as a way of telling them, "Don't bother your father," and they went about their business as if I wasn't there.

I sighed in defeat. I knew I had to maintain a strict regimen of exercise and healthy eating. No more excuses. No more cheating. Lois left to take the children to school. I showered, dressed, and headed off to work.

When I got home that night, Lois was all smiles. "Honey, I swung by the bookstore today and got some great cookbooks! I'm making a dinner tonight I know you'll enjoy."

I refused to be encouraged, "What about the kids. They won't want to eat diabetic food." My daughter Lisa was beginning to miss pepperoni.

She laughed, "Not to worry. They're going out for pizza with my sister. It'll just be you and me tonight."

She was really excited about the meal, so I tried to be more upbeat. Lois was known for her great cooking. She went on talking about the cookbooks and how she was looking forward to learning more about portion control and finding foods that were better for my blood sugar levels.

I set the table while she finished cooking. When we sat down to a meal of baked fish, I immediately noticed the smaller portions and all the vegetables. I sat in silence for a few minutes, thinking about how I had been raised in a "meat and potatoes" family. I loved baked potatoes dripping in butter and sour cream – I mean, who doesn't? I also enjoyed thick, juicy steaks, and cheese bread. Not every day, but...

I kept the conversation on topics unrelated to food, hoping she wouldn't notice how hard it was for me to clean my plate.

But finally, as we cleared the table Lois asked, "How was your dinner?"

"Good, honey." I fibbed. I put my arms around her and kissed her forehead. "Thank you for being on my side."

She smiled, "I'm always on your side, Joe." She glanced up at the clock and turned toward the sink.

"I'll clean up the kitchen and you can get in your walk before sundown."

Her words felt like a cold slap in the face. I thought to myself, I'm tired of being reminded that I need to exercise! Before I could stop myself I said, "I don't need you to tell me when to walk or not!"

She glanced at me with a hurt look on her face. "Joe, I'm trying to help you. That's why I went to the trouble of cooking this meal."

Slipping into a downward spiral of emotions, I blurted out, "Everything about my life is trouble right now, Lois. I don't like the food I have to eat. I don't like having to walk every day. And it doesn't help that you're nagging me about it."

She turned back to the sink. "I'm trying to be supportive and you call that nagging? You've been so hard to live with ever since you received your diagnosis. Your condition doesn't just affect you, Joe. It impacts all of us!"

"Great! Now I'm the bad guy." I was so frustrated I left the room. I wouldn't admit to Lois that I'd already intended to walk that evening. If I went out now, it would seem like I was buckling to her pressure. Instead, I sat down at my computer to check my email.

I scanned down my inbox and saw one from my cousin, Randy, telling me about a family reunion set for next summer. You've got to be kidding, I thought to myself as I read over the email. They're planning a family hike through the Smokey

Mountains. I won't be in shape for that. And there's no way I'm telling them that I have diabetes. It's too humiliating.

The phone rang.

It was Rob, once again asking me to sub for the bowling league. I asked, "When do you need a player?"

"Tonight, Joe."

"What?"

"I know its short notice, but I just got a call from Greg and he's stuck at the office. We need you to come down here so we can stay in the league."

Any excuse for being out of the house tonight after this run-in with Lois sounded good. "Okay, Rob. I'll be right down."

I grabbed my jacket, keys, and headed out the back door. "Rob and the guys need me to sub at the bowling league tonight. Don't wait up."

Lois didn't respond, but I noticed that the kitchen was especially clean. She always cleans when she's upset.

The time at the bowling alley didn't turn out much better than dinner. My buddies were already on their second or third beers, happily munching on burgers and fries. Even though I'd just had dinner, I was still hungry so I ordered a wimpy salad and diet cola. One of the guys laughed and said, "Hey guys. Check out what poor Joe's having for dinner!"

Rob looked over at me, but didn't say anything about my diabetes. I laughed along with them. I hadn't told any of them, except Rob, about my diabetes. I said, "Don't worry. I'm just warming up." Then I ordered a Sloppy Joe, onion rings, and a beer. I felt like a kid in high school trying to fit in. But I figured, after that paltry dinner at home, I deserve something good to eat.

It was late when I got home, so I skipped taking my blood sugar. But in the morning, my blood glucose was way back up. I didn't tell Lois what my numbers were and she didn't ask. But I knew I couldn't keep this up.

I felt guilty and frustrated with myself.

On the way to work I made a tough decision.

During a break I called my doctor's office. I told the nurse that I was finally willing to take medication. She said that she'd have the doctor call over a prescription. Now maybe I can get my life back to normal, I thought. All I need is a little magic pill.

While part of me felt like I had given in, another part of me was relieved to have asked for help.

Someone... Please Fix My Problem!

The next two weeks were drudgery. Every meal was unpleasant—an experience of deprivation and crumbling willpower. I forced myself to walk every evening or at least most evenings. I resented every single step.

Lois no longer tried to help me, which meant that she didn't push me to attend the class. We came to an unspoken arrangement that talking about my diabetes was off limits – at least for now.

By the time the next class rolled around, I was anything but hopeful. But I had nothing to lose at this point. Maybe I'd learn something new. At the very least, I could hang out with others facing diabetes and not feel so alone.

I arrived right as the class started. Even though I saw Ram had an empty seat next to him, I sat towards the back without making eye contact with anyone else. I didn't want to talk to anybody. As I looked around, I saw a few new faces, but most were the familiar ones from the first week.

Marianne started the class with her usual bright smile. I thought to myself, how can she seem so happy when she's got to be as miserable as I am?

She welcomed everyone and began, "In our last class, we talked about SARAH (Shock, Surprise or Sadness; Anger; Rationalization; Acceptance; and Help or Hope) and, very importantly, the Dreaded Drama Triangle, or DDT. The dynamics between the roles of Victim, Persecutor, and Rescuer take place in a very particular Orientation.[1]

---

1   A grateful heartfelt "thank you" to Bob Anderson, founder of The Leadership Circle, for introducing David to the concept and graphic depiction of the life orientations and pattern of results they produce and his support of this adaptation that appear in the next few chapters. To learn more about these models, see his White Papers under the Resources section of www.theleadershipcircle.com.

"Tonight I want to first introduce you to what I mean by an Orientation, which will give us a way to consider how we view and react to our diabetes.

"The way that we look at the world is our Orientation. It defines how we view ourselves, how we orient ourselves toward everything and everyone around us. And it has a great deal to do with what shows up in our life experience.

"Here's the way we frame an Orientation—it's called the FISBE." Marianne drew three large circles on the board. In the top circle she wrote, *Focus* and drew an arrow from that circle to the one below it to the right. In the second circle, she wrote *Inner State* with another arrow to the third circle. Finally, she wrote *Behavior* in the last circle and completed the cycle by drawing a third arrow back to the top circle.

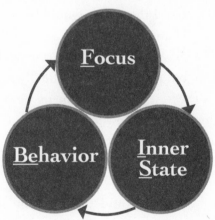

"If we underline the first letters of each term we have FISBE. What we *F*ocus on, or think about, engages an *I*nner *S*tate, which is our emotional response. Those feelings then drive our *Be*havior."

"Now let's apply the FISBE Orientation model to how we view our diabetes.

"How many here have received your diagnosis in the last three months?" A few hands went up.

"How many in the last 3-6 months?" About half the hands went up, including mine.

"How many more than 6 months ago?" The rest of the hands went up.

One man spoke up, "How about more than 3 years? I pretty much ignored my symptoms and the doctor's advice until I started having trouble with my kidneys. That got my attention big time. My kidneys are overworked trying to manage the high blood sugar. It's pretty serious. Since then I have been trying to work with my diabetes, but it has been harder than I thought it would be."

She said, "Thanks for being so candid. Obviously, the sooner we get off the roller coaster the better in the long run, but the fact that you finally faced your situation is the key. Thanks for being here."

Marianne then turned to the class, "I feel safe in guessing that many of you have tried following some kind of plan, but have had less than sustainable success."

Heads bobbed up and down. Someone murmured, "You got that right."

"I know what you've been through because that's how I started my journey with diabetes,"

Marianne admitted. "I want to share something with you and see if it describes how these months have been for you."

She swept her eyes across the whole room. "When I first received my diagnosis and began grappling with the realities of diabetes, I did so from a problem-focused and reactive way of seeing my disease. It was from what I call the Victim Orientation."

She turned back to the board and drew another three-circle diagram.

She said, "When I was first diagnosed, I definitely looked at my diabetes as a problem." In the top circle she wrote the word *Problem*. "In my mind, I had a problem that was turning my world upside down—diabetes. It definitely was my Focus."

A woman in her sixties raised her hand, "Diabetes IS a problem. It's ruining my life." Others nodded in agreement and a man near me said, "Mine too!" I think we all shared that sentiment.

Marianne nodded, "Well, let's explore what that means for you. If you focus on diabetes as a problem, then how do you feel?"

"Frightened," said one person.

"Overwhelmed," said another.

"Confused," said someone else.

Marianne wrote *Anxiety* in the second circle. "All of the feelings you have identified are anxiety or fear based, and so that's how we label the Inner State. There are many forms and differing intensities of anxiety.

"This Inner State of anxiety then drives our <u>Be</u>havior, which is reactive in nature. We react to the anxiety we are feeling about the problem," Marianne said as she wrote *React* in the last circle.

Victim Orientation

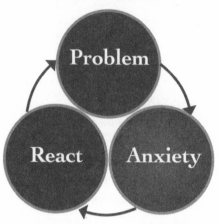

She then asked us, "How have you reacted to the anxiety you have felt, or are still feeling, about your diabetes?"

A man dressed in running clothes said, "I become determined to tackle this disease!"

Marianne pointed to a woman up front, "How do you react?"

She said, "I feel paralyzed. I don't know what to do."

Marianne asked, "Do any of you try to pretend it isn't happening to you or hope it will just go away?" A few people nodded.

"What you have described are the three typical ways people respond to problems. We fight, freeze or flee." She paused. "And we usually, at one time or another, do all three."

I thought to myself, has Marianne been following me around? She described me perfectly. Since my diagnosis, I have naively thought I could fight it by learning about the disease, exercising, and eating right. But when things haven't progress as I expected they would, I freeze up. The more anxious I become, the more I minimize its importance and want to run away.

Marianne said, "When we define diabetes as a problem, our attention is focused on what we *don't want* and *don't like*: the disease. This raises our anxiety, which moves us to action. Our intention then becomes a frantic effort to get rid of, or away from, the disease.

"Repeatedly focusing on a problem, engaging inner anxiety, and reacting, actually produces a predictable pattern of results I call the roller coaster."

She then drew a diagram on the whiteboard:

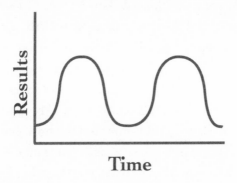

I smiled to myself, Ah, yes. The roller coaster. I know it well.

As she drew, Marianne said, "As anxiety gets engaged, we react and, over time, the results get better. Now, you might think that experiencing positive results would motivate us to keep up our new behaviors, but, ironically, that's not the case. When we experience positive results, our anxiety decreases because of the improvement. And when we're less anxious, we actually lose our energy for action. We typically go back to old habits and patterns."

As Marianne drew the rising and falling line, I realized that I had followed this same pattern exactly. She said, "This is how we end up riding the roller coaster of action and inaction, of working diligently and slacking off."

Nailed me again! I thought.

"Here is an example that all too many of us in this room can relate to. It has to do with the cycle of weight gain and loss. When I step on the scale in the morning I feel some *anxiety* over the number of pounds that I see. I *react* by promising myself to diet and exercise. I stay focused and committed for a while. I start to lose pounds and inches and, pretty soon, I'm feeling really great. My clothes fit better. My friends and family tell me how good I'm looking. My results – less weight – are increasing.

"But then something comes up, like a big holiday or a vacation. Since my anxiety has decreased because of the results of looking and feeling good, as well as feeling a bit deprived, I celebrate by eating all the things I've been avoiding. I tell myself it is just for a while anyway. I'll get back to eating healthy again soon. But since I feel like I deserve a reward, and I'm not anxious anymore, I start to gain weight again. Before I know it, I'm standing on the same scale on a whole new morning wondering how all those problem pounds came back. Sound familiar?" she asked.

I let out a big sigh of relief. Finally I'd found someone who understood what I'd been going through. I've been fighting, fleeing, and freezing. I'd fight for a while, see a few positive results and then slip back into poaching a piece of pizza here, snatching a piece of candy there, and rationalizing that I had exercised enough for the week.

"Just a couple of additional points for this evening," she said. "First, it is important to understand how anxiety plays a central role in this mind-set. Do you see how it really drives this whole system? As long as anxiety is high, you have energy for action, or rather, reaction.

"Let's connect the Dreaded Drama Triangle together with Victim Orientation FISBE. All three roles in the DDT – the Victim, Persecutor, and Rescuer – are reactive in nature. A big part of what moves us around the triangle and causes us to take different roles is that one person reacts and then the others in the drama react to those reactions – and off we all go! All the players focus on each other as 'problems.' This triggers our Inner State (emotional responses) which is reflected in our behavior. We end up reacting to reactions. It is *very* difficult to break the cycle."

Marianne paused and looked at her watch. "But let's not end there. Are you up for a more hopeful and empowered relationship with your disease?"

"Sure." "You bet." "I'd love it" and similar responses were heard around the room.

Marianne said, "Before we end our class tonight, I want to give you some homework. For the next two weeks, observe whether or not you are riding the roller coaster."

Marianne asked for questions or comments. I blurted out, "Is there a more effective Orientation to our diabetes that gets us out of the DDT patterns?"

She smiled, "That's a great question and the short answer is 'yes.' We will definitely move into that in the next class. For now, I want you to just pay attention to how you are reacting to your diabetes between now and next week.

"That's it for class tonight, folks. I look forward to seeing you again at our next meeting."

I gathered my things, but didn't head out immediately to my car. Still immersed in my thoughts, I watched as people chatted and got better acquainted.

I then walked up to the front of the room where Ram was sitting. He had struck up a conversation with a woman who had sat next to him. He said, "We all seemed pretty discouraged by that Victim Orientation tonight."

The woman nodded her head. "I feel doomed to repeat the drama, riding the roller coaster of progress and setbacks. I hope Marianne gives us something substantial next session that we can actually use." She grinned, "I like insight into my dysfunction as well as the next gal, but I need help that works in my life on a daily basis."

I came out of my fog and joined in, "Yeah. If my doctor isn't going to give me an answer other than exercise more, eat right, and take medication, then what will I do? I don't want to go back and have him hassle me about failing. I don't see a way out of this. I wish I could find a more supportive doctor."

"That reminds me," the woman said, "I was given this card by someone else in the class tonight. Maybe this new doctor could help us both." She started looking through her purse.

I asked, "What's his name – maybe he is in my network."

"It's not a he," she said, finally locating the card. "Here it is. Her name is Dr. Theresa Elizabeth Davis. The person that gave it to me referred to her as Doctor Ted. That's interesting, it even says under her name 'Dr. Ted.'," she said handing me the card. "Write down her info. I'm going to see if I can get an appointment as soon as possible. I'm not happy with what I'm receiving from my doctor either."

I brought out my notebook and pen and copied down Dr. Ted's phone number. As I wrote it down, I said, "Thank you! Maybe Dr. Ted can point me in a healthy direction. I'll call her tomorrow." I was really hoping that Dr. Ted would provide the help I needed.

CHAPTER

FOUR

Straight-shooters by My Side

Even though I wasn't overly hopeful the next morning, I checked out Dr. Ted. What have I got to lose? I asked myself, and went online to see if she was in my insurance carrier's network. Sure enough, her name was there, so I gave her office a call.

She was a busy doctor. Luckily, they had just received a cancellation for the following week. The receptionist asked me if I had an email address so she could send me some information, which I thought was a bit odd. I gave it to her and within an hour I had an email from Dr. Ted's office that welcomed me and included forms for me to fill out, including one which gave them permission to request my records from my current doctor.

The email also informed me that an order was already submitted to their clinic's lab for my blood to be drawn, along with the address for the lab and a map with directions. I knew then that this was going to be a different kind of doctor. It felt good to be doing something proactive.

In the meantime, all I knew to do was what I'd done before — exercise, be careful about what I ate, and watch my numbers. It was easy to fall back into a pattern of rewarding myself with some sort of a treat when my numbers were low. Of course, my numbers went back up after such an indulgence. How miserable my life had become. In fact, I felt even more discouraged than before. Now that I had learned all about SARAH, DDT, FISBE, the Victim Orientation, and its roller coaster, I could see all of the mistakes I was making. But I didn't know what else to do.

Over the next few days I returned all the forms and had my blood taken. On the day of the appointment I arrived a bit early at Dr. Ted's office. No doubt I'll have to wait a while, I thought to myself. I guess I was a bit excited to meet with a doctor who might do more than scold me.

After I checked in at the front desk, I found a seat in an attractively decorated lobby. Rather than being holed up in a small, crowded waiting room, Dr. Ted provided her patients with an area filled with green plants and natural light. A fountain bubbled in the background. As I scanned the other patients, there were many people who looked healthy and hopeful. I thought, this is quite a change from what I'm used to with my other doctor.

Before long, I heard my name called and I followed a young man, who introduced himself as Carson, back into the hallway.

Carson pointed me into an exam room and smiled, "So this is your first visit with us?"

"Yes." I said.

"Good. Welcome. I'll begin by taking your vital signs, weight, and all. Then you'll meet with our Diabetes Educator for a few minutes. She can fill you in on the way we do things here before you meet with Dr. Ted."

As Carson wrapped the blood pressure cuff around my arm, I noticed a few posters around the room. Rather than the usual "Warning" posters I usually saw in doctors' offices, the information was positive and encouraging. One poster caught my eye. It said "To the Creator in you!" It had a diagram with three circles, just like the ones used in Marianne's class, but this one was labeled "Creator Orientation." None of the terms made much sense to me at the time. I said, "I don't know what that means, but it's nice to see positive information rather than the usual scare tactics."

Carson smiled, "I hear that a lot from first time patients. We have a unique way of working with patients who have diabetes. I love being a part of something healing."

After he finished writing my results in the chart, Carson led me into another office to meet with the Diabetes Educator. Imagine my surprise when I was introduced to Marianne, the instructor at my class!

She shook my hand and said, "I recognize you. You're rather new to the Monday night class, aren't you?"

I smiled and nodded. I was delighted to get to work with her on an individual basis.

She told me, "I am careful not to promote Dr. Ted too early during the classes at the community center, even though the seminar is based on her essential principles. I teach a similar class here at the clinic on the alternate weeks. I was so fortunate to discover Dr. Ted when I was diagnosed with diabetes. I was inspired by her approach, so I decided to spread the word through my classes, along with the work I do with patients here."

I noticed that the same two posters were in her office. I pointed to the Creator Orientation diagram and asked, "Can I expect to see those in an upcoming class?"

Marianne smiled, "Oh, yes. Your diabetes will really take on new meaning when you become a Creator. Adopting a Creator Orientation is the topic of the next class. You've already made it through the 'downer' part of the curriculum."

I moaned, "I'm glad to hear that!"

Marianne smiled, "I am confident you are going to find this Orientation a fundamental change in how you approach your diabetes, something that Dr. Ted will share with you briefly today."

"Sounds good. My experience with diabetes has definitely been difficult," I agreed.

Marianne looked at my chart, "Let's take a look at your labs. While your numbers are indicators of how things have been going, focusing solely on them tends to reinforce the Victim Orientation. Usually a person's anxiety goes up as the numbers go up and diminishes as the numbers go down, just like the roller coaster pattern we talked about in class. They are important to track, but they are not the primary place to put your focus."

I told her, "My numbers were all my previous doctor cared about."

Marianne explained that she would always meet with me before the doctor in order to help me prepare for my session with Dr. Ted. "She really encourages you to ask questions and to be actively involved in your treatment. We have noticed that passive patients are much more likely to want their doctor to be a Rescuer." Wrapping up, Marianne stood and said, "I'll let Dr. Ted know that you're here and ready to meet with her. I will see you at the next class."

Hello Dr. Ted

Marianne left and I thumbed through a health magazine. I was very curious to learn more about this Creator stuff. Before long, I heard a firm tap on the door and Dr. Ted entered the room. I was immediately put at ease by her warm handshake and caring eyes that looked at me over a pair of reading glasses perched on her nose. "Good to meet you, Joe. I'm Dr. Ted."

Petite and slender, Dr. Ted appeared to be in her late 50s or early 60s. Her salt-and-pepper hair was wrapped up on top of her head. She was clearly energized by her work, giving me the sense that she had all the time in the world for me.

She looked at my chart and said, "I understand from Marianne that you are attending the class series at the community center. That's great, Joe! It is impossible to see your doctor for fifteen minutes four to six times a year and expect them to teach you all that you need to know about diabetes and how to live effectively with it. I also know the class just covered the Victim Orientation, which I am confident will not be the way you relate to your condition in the long run.

"If you choose to be a patient of ours, we will be supporting you in adopting a Creator Orientation. We stress being proactive in living a meaningful and fulfilling life with diabetes, rather than simply reacting to it. We believe very deeply in health empowerment for our patients. In this mind-set, your focus is actually not on the diabetes itself; it is on creating a life of meaning and purpose, including optimal health for yourself. We want you to go after whatever is on your bucket list."

"What do you mean, my bucket list?"

Dr. Ted smiled broadly, "That's a term I learned from a movie several years back. It's all those things you want to do and to experience in your life before you – if you will excuse the expression – 'kick the bucket'."

"You mean die?"

"Yes, Joe, we all will die eventually. If you learn to deal with your diabetes from a Creator Orientation and take the steps necessary to live a healthy life, there is no reason to doubt that you can live a life of meaning, fulfillment, and vitality. Is that something you would like – to live a healthy life so you can go after your bucket list?" she asked sincerely.

I thought for a moment and said, "Sure. But with the onset of diabetes that doesn't seem possible." I lapsed into sarcasm. "I mean, since I have diabetes, aren't I going to go blind, lose a limb, have kidney failure, a stroke, or a heart attack? It doesn't seem to be that much of a future."

"I certainly won't lie to you, Joe. It is true that diabetes has the potential to shorten life or to lessen the quality of life – but that's not a certainty. That's definitely not a defined future for you. If you keep your numbers in range – as a measure of how you are managing your health – then I believe that you will lead a long and fulfilling life. The challenge is to learn how to create an enjoyable lifestyle that is healthy at the same time!"

I laughed, "Well, if you put it that way, it does make sense. Who says being healthy can't be enjoyable?"

She nodded. "Over time you will be surprised, Joe, at how your quality of life will improve. Take a look at this diagram. It follows the same FISBE pattern that Marianne presents in the class.

Creator Orientation

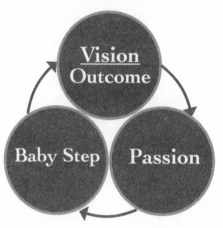

"At the top you see the words *Vision* and *Outcome*, which is where you put your focus. If you choose to pursue health as your envisioned outcome, and if it is an outcome you really care about, you'll tap into the inner state of *Passion* and desire for an ongoing state of health.

"Propelled by that passion, you will develop new habits and behaviors that include all the necessary Baby Steps for you to grow into and come to own your health and well-being, even given the challenge that diabetes presents.

"Instead of trying to get away from or get rid of your diabetes, you will focus on what you *do* want

– which is health, vitality, wellbeing – even greater peace-of-mind. Rather than define yourself as a diabetic, you will see yourself as a person with diabetes. There's a significant difference in these two perspectives."

I responded, "Health and wellbeing sound good to me. I really do want that for my life. I have a lot left on bucket list!"

"Good!" Dr. Ted smiled. "Then I am confident we can work together."

She then looked at the chart on her clipboard and said, "I am glad to see that you are currently taking medication. Are you taking it as prescribed, both morning and at night?"

"Most of the time. I forget sometimes at night."

"What can you do to create a reminder?"

"Hmm…" I thought aloud. "Maybe set the alarm on my phone to go off at a particular time?"

"That sounds perfect. Just make sure you eat a little something, maybe a small bowl of low-fat cottage cheese, when you take it. This medication is best taken with some food, or else your stomach might feel a little queasy. Now tell me, what else are you doing to take care of yourself?"

"The usual," I said, looking a bit forlorn. "Exercise and watching what I eat."

"Are you tracking your glucose?"

"Most of the time. OK, to tell the truth, some of the time. I get tired of pricking my finger several times a day."

Dr. Ted sat down on the stool across from me and looked me straight in the eye. "I want to thank you and reinforce something that you just did. You initially started to shade the truth on measuring your glucose, but then decided to be honest. As we work together as partners to create optimal health in your life, it is absolutely imperative that you always tell me the truth – even if it is not pleasant. If I don't know your current reality, I cannot effectively coach or challenge you. I promise I will not judge you, but I will hold you accountable for commitments and actions you take or don't take. Fair enough?"

"Fair enough." I liked this straight-shooter.

She said, "Let me take a minute to explain what is going on in your body. When you eat, your food is broken down into three sources of energy: protein, sugar, and fats. One of the jobs of your pancreas is to make sure you have just the right amount of sugar in your blood stream so your body can use it.

"If your blood sugar gets too low, it's called hypoglycemia. You might feel nervous. Your heart might speed up. Your vision can blur, and you might even pass out. In severe cases, a person could go into a coma or even die. Also, when your blood sugar is too low, your pancreas breaks down glycogen in your liver into glucose and releases it into the blood."

I said, "Sounds like keeping the right level of sugar in my blood is pretty important!"

"Absolutely." Dr. Ted nodded. "It's also critical that your blood sugar doesn't get too high.

"I see from your chart that you report that you urinate often. Let me explain why that is. Once your blood sugar gets too high, your kidneys cannot reabsorb the glucose from the urine and so it passes and pulls water from your body. The higher the glucose, the more the water that is pulled out. Eventually it leads to significant water loss."

"Hmm. I actually think I understand that." I said.

"This is where high blood sugar and insulin comes in. Your pancreas secretes insulin to trigger your body to pull sugar out of your blood and to store it for energy or for later. Without a proper level of insulin, you soon suffer the impact of high blood sugar — possible nerve damage, heart disease, kidney, and eye problems."

I nodded. "Yes, I know. All of those scary things I've been reading about."

She continued, "Joe, you can't rely on your pancreas to perform its duties like you have in the past. It's now up to you to help regulate the amount of sugar in your blood. That's why it's so important for you to be aware of what you are eating. If you eat too much food that turns into sugar, you will stress out your system. Exercise helps lower blood sugar as well, because you are burning up the sugar as energy."

I joked, "So you're not just trying to make my life miserable for the fun of it?"

"No. I'm not trying to make your life miserable at all," she smiled. "I'm empowering you to take responsibility and to make choices to enhance your health and well-being."

"It's beginning to make sense to me now. You know, why diet and exercise are so important. I haven't felt this positive since before my diagnosis." I told her.

She smiled again, "You're becoming what we call an 'activated patient.'"

I laughed, "Well, that's exactly how I feel... activated!"

One Step Forward...

I left her office with a lightness of heart and a new vision of health, rather than feeling victimized by my diabetes. And I was really looking forward to my next class with Marianne. I wanted to learn all I could about this Creator Orientation. For the first time, I actually felt there was a possibility of living a long rewarding life, even with my diabetes.

When I got home, I shared what I'd learned from Dr. Ted with Lois. "If it will make you easier to live with," Lois told me, "I'm all for it."

I answered. "That's fair! Each time I've gotten a burst of encouragement, I've soon fallen flat. That roller coaster ride has gotten old for all of us. I sure hope this time will be different. At least it looks good on paper!"

During the following week, I followed Dr. Ted's advice as close as I could. I set my phone alarm to go off at 7:00 each morning and night to remind me to take my medication just before I ate. I spent time looking up websites on nutrition. Portion control was a big theme that I saw over and over again. I also checked out the labels on some of the foods we were eating. I was amazed at how many of the things we regularly ate, even those that claimed to be "natural" and "healthy," were high in fat, calories, and carbs. No wonder my blood sugar had been so hard to regulate. Even when I thought I was eating well, I was consuming a lot that was damaging to my health.

Then day-to-day life once again intruded. As in the past, it wasn't long before I lost interest in this level of effort and wanted my old life back. I just didn't want to accept that life as I once knew it was over. Whatever I did one day reflected in my blood sugar numbers the next. When I exercised and ate healthy food, my numbers inched downward. When I lapsed back into my old patterns, the numbers would climb back beyond safe levels.

The night before my next class, Lois and I were settling into bed. As Lois reached to turn off the light, I said "I really need to go to this class tomorrow. I need another boost to keep on track."

She put her head on my shoulder and sighed, "Joe, I'm proud of all the effort you are putting into this. I know this must be very hard for you. But, you know, it's been hard on the kids and me too. No sugar in the house, no soft drinks, no white bread, no more doughnuts, rarely any ice cream. It's no longer a fun place."

"I was hoping for more encouragement than that, Lois."

"Well, you act as if this disease is all about you. It's not. It would help if you were more encouraging to me and the kids as well. We're not here just to make sure you get through the day."

I grunted and flopped my head on the pillow. "Kick a guy when he's down."

Lois turned off the light. "No one can get you off the floor but yourself. I'm tired of all this."

I reached over and pulled Lois close to me. "Don't give up on me, honey." I kissed her on the top of her head. "I know I can be self-focused and forget that we're in this together."

She leaned up and kissed me on the cheek. "I'm not. Really, I'm not. I just don't know how to help you...to help all of us cope with this change."

"I know, Lois. And I really appreciate your effort. We'll figure this out together. Dr. Ted and Marianne have given me a glimpse of a better way of living."

Lois leaned back on her pillow. "Well, we're all hoping that they have more tools up their sleeves than we've seen so far."

Lois soon fell asleep, but my head swirled with worry. Lois was right about my self-focus. My numbers were up and down, up and down and so was I - on an emotional level. I gained hope when I talked with people at the class or Marianne or Dr. Ted. But all too soon, I felt angry and resentful that I had diabetes.

Is this the most I can expect from life, now? I go to a class or a doctor's appointment and get a pep talk from these people and think dealing with diabetes is doable, only to flop once I face day-to-day reality? If that's the case, I'll need to go to a class everyday! How pathetic is that?

I was further annoyed by having to get up and go to the bathroom again. It was quite a while before I finally fell into a fretful sleep.

CHAPTER

FIVE

Gratitude or Attitude?

I was relieved when the next class came around. I walked into the room, glad to see Ram and the woman we'd talked to during the last class.

As I walked up the woman asked, "Did you see Dr. Ted?"

"Yes, I did. She's amazing!" I exclaimed.

"I should have followed through too. I put it off and ended up meeting with my regular doctor," she confessed. "I thought since my doctor is a woman, it would turn out okay. During the appointment, she referred to me as a diabetic. Without thinking, I just let her have it! Doctors can sure dish out criticism, but I don't think they like conflict or push-back from assertive patients sometimes."

She chuckled. "I said to her, 'I am a person with diabetes, NOT a diabetic.' My doctor's mouth dropped and I just kept going. I said, 'How would you like it if I called you a morbid 'obesitetic' just because you are overweight?' I just made that word up on the spot."

By now, Ram and I both grinned. I asked, "So what did she say?"

"She just sputtered and abruptly left the room. Looking back, I felt victimized by her and then took on the role of Persecutor when I told her off. I tracked her down in her office and apologized. She waved me off. By that point, we were both embarrassed."

Ram leaned over and nudged her. "Good for you and great insight on the DDT roles! It is a challenge to see myself as a Persecutor. It's easier to feel like a Victim in this experience."

She shook her head. "Well, I've got to learn how to do that without being so rude to other people. I'll bet you she never calls me a diabetic again!"

I laughed, "I bet she's been cured!"

Ram looked around and pointed out that there were a lot of new faces in the room.

Marianne's voice called us to order. We all turned around to face the front.

Marianne said, "You might have noticed that our class is larger than last time. A number of the graduates of this course attend an alumni group that you are all invited to join after our last class together. A number of the alumni like to attend some of my classes as reminders and refreshers – and to give me support."

She looked over to the alumni group members and said, "You don't need me to speak for you.

Would any of you like to share why you're in attendance tonight?"

A man spoke up, "Hi everyone, my name is Mark. I'd be glad to say why I'm here." Addressing the group he said, "I try to attend the third class in Marianne's series as often as I can. I never get tired of watching the light bulbs come on for folks when they learn about adopting a Creator Orientation.

"This was the beginning of great success for me," he continued. "It is kind of like riding a bike. You can read all the books you want, but it is not until you get on and actually ride and learn to balance that you gain the skill and mastery over it.

"Over time, you ride without even having to think about it. Once you learn to ride – and to approach your diabetes from this mind-set – your life will never be the same again." He smiled broadly and sat down.

Then a woman spoke up, "I came here tonight to give you all encouragement. I remember how I felt after the second class and I needed the extra support. So, I'm here to tell you--don't give up! Hearing about taking on a Creator Orientation and actually living it are very different experiences. I think you'll get a much better picture of what this is all about in tonight's class."

Their supportive and optimistic words were uplifting to hear. I thought, I sure hope so. I'm tired of being disappointed by the ideas that seem so good when I learn about them. I guess I'm really disappointed in myself.

Another woman chimed in, "I also enjoy seeing how the information in this class helps people to gain new hope. As I look back over all the changes that have come into my life, I can honestly say that I have come to be grateful for my diagnosis. It really got my attention."

Her comment stopped me short. I thought, she's grateful for her diagnosis? You've got to be kidding! I can't imagine ever being grateful for having this disease.

She stood up as she grew even more excited, "If I had not developed diabetes, which I have learned is a condition that can be managed, it could have been a heart attack or a stroke that got my attention and that would have been even harder to deal with. Looking back, I realize that I was living an unhealthy lifestyle and yet pretended everything was OK because I didn't feel sick... yet.

"Don't confuse not feeling sick with being healthy, my friends. I now know I am healthy because of what I learned here. My new lifestyle and all these numbers we have become aware of confirm that. I feel great these days. For me, diabetes was that wake-up call I needed to begin to live my life on purpose." She laughed and began to sit down. "That's the end of my sermon and testimony – for now."

Marianne thanked the guests for sharing and turned to the class. "I'd like to start off tonight by hearing from you. Did you see the Victim Orientation and DDT in action in your lives this week?"

A woman in the back of the room spoke up, "I saw how DDT applies to my entire life, not just diabetes. I saw myself flipping among the roles of Victim, Rescuer, and Persecutor at work and at home. No matter which role I was in, I could see that they were all reactions to problems in my life."

A young man said, "I saw a number of ways that I reacted, but the biggest Persecutor in my life this week was played by my doctor. I'm so frustrated with the way he and his staff treat me. Sorry to say that, but you asked us to be candid in this class."

Marianne said, "This model does expose those in the medical profession that see diabetes – or any other disease, for that matter – as a problem to solve, rather than an opportunity to empower patients to take responsibility for their own health."

The woman Ram and I had been talking with before class spoke up, "I confronted my doctor this week. Perhaps not in the kindest of ways, but I was really irritated by her attitude."

"It's easy to feel let down while gaining new insight," Marianne affirmed. "After all, we've been led to believe that the medical community will somehow rescue us."

A Breath of Fresh AIR

Marianne continued, "For tonight, I want to stress that, unlike a Rescuer who sees you all as Victims who are powerless to care for yourselves, I see each and every one of you as capable, resourceful, and empowered. Whether you realize your personal power yet or not, I am here to support you in creating outcomes in your lives – including health and well-being. In order to do so, however, it requires that you replace the problem focused Victim Orientation with a Creator Orientation.

Marianne then presented to the class the Creator Orientation FISBE model that I had seen at Dr. Ted's office. She explained how a focus on vision and outcomes taps into passion that then drives the behavior of taking Baby Steps in creating the outcome.

"Now that we see these two different Orientations," she said, "Tonight I want to focus on three key distinctions between the two orientations."

She wrote on the whiteboard the following letters:

A

I

R

"We use AIR because, as you will see, these two orientations and life stances have very different characteristics or 'airs' about them." Several people chuckled, but I was more perplexed than amused.

She continued, "The first distinction has to do with where we put our *Attention*. If you remember from two classes ago, in the Victim Orientation our attention is focused on *what we don't want* and *don't like* – which is why we call them problems. I think it is fair to say that all of us don't want or like diabetes, right?"

No kidding, I thought.

"When we adopt a Creator Orientation, our attention is on what we *do want* and what we *do like* – for instance, health and well-being. There is a very different quality of attention that results when we focus on what we want.

"It is like being on a diet. If you think about what you are not going to eat all day, it will drive you crazy. If you focus on what you do intend to eat and go find ways to do this, then it feels completely different.

"Can you feel the difference between my saying 'I don't want or like diabetes' compared to 'I choose to live a healthy and fulfilling life with diabetes?'" Marianne asked.

Mark from the alumni group spoke up, "Marianne, I'd like to quickly add that my choosing and living a vital lifestyle has enlarged my view of my whole life. Rather than narrowing in on one part of my health, I see the larger picture of living a full and meaningful life."

"Indeed, it makes a world of difference," Marianne affirmed. "The second difference – the *I* in AIR – is in our *Intention*. I want you to recall the FISBE of the Victim Orientation. In that mind-set, what is the Focus on?"

The woman behind me said, "I focus on my problems."

Marianne nodded. "And what is your Inner State?"

Someone from the back said, "I am scared and anxious."

Another man said, "I just shut down completely. I feel overwhelmed."

Marianne continued, "That leads me to the last question. What behavior comes from anxiety?"

I knew the answer to that one. "I react. I am not intentional. I feel controlled by the situation, like my mind makes up all these stories about all the bad things that are going to happen to me."

One of the women from the alumni group said aloud, "I just love this class!"

I laughed to myself. I had to admit that these folks were a boost to my mood. Hearing other people say out loud what I was thinking and feeling, plus seeing all the confidence from them and the staff at Dr. Ted's, was exciting and made me feel better.

Marianne continued, "Good! So, in the Victim Orientation, our Intention is to *get rid of or away from…* what?"

"The problem!" several people said in unison.

Marianne put up her hand. "Well, actually, this is a little bit of a trick question. You are right, we tell ourselves that it is to get rid of the problem. The real intention here is to get rid of – or move away from – our inner state of anxiety.

"It may be true that, if we *are* able to solve the problem, perhaps the anxiety will go away. But if we don't or can't eliminate the problem, we will take action – we will react – to the anxiety. As we also talked about previously, the three primary ways in which we do this are fight, flight, or freeze."

The woman behind us said, "I think I do all three simultaneously!"

A chuckle moved through the group.

"Now," Marianne paused. "Let's take a look at the Creator Orientation. As a Creator, our Intention is to *move toward and bring into being* our envisioned outcome. So the key difference about Intention between the Orientations is that of moving away from the problem versus moving toward the desired outcome."

I thought to myself, this is making more sense to me now.

Marianne continued, "Last, but not least, these two orientations lead to two very different patterns of Results that emerge over time. So, the R in AIR is for *Results*." Marianne drew:

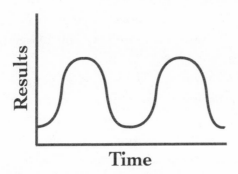

Then asked, "Does this look familiar?"

I spoke up, "That's the roller coaster ride of the Victim Orientation. I know that one very well."

"Right you are! Now we will see a very different pattern of results that emerge over time as we live our lives from a Creator Orientation. To see how the pattern surfaces, let's look at the relationship between the components of the FISBE.

"As you focus on an envisioned outcome – like a vital, healthy, and meaningful life – what happens to your passion? Does it increase or diminish?"

I answered, "It increases."

Marianne asked me, "If your passion and desire increases, what then happens to your tendency to take Baby Step actions or engage in healthy behaviors?"

"It grows." I said.

"The passion or desire motivates you to take action - to take Baby Steps, which is the Behavior, or action, you take in a Creator Orientation. With each step, you get closer to – or become clearer about – your outcome. As you move toward your vision, your passion increases, you take Baby Steps and, over time, you get closer and closer to your outcome.

"However, every Baby Step is not necessarily forward progress. Sometimes we make mistakes or take a step that seems to move us farther away from our goal or envisioned outcomes. The good news is that, from this Creator mind-set, even mistakes or steps back can provide important learning for how we move forward. That's why we say that every step gets us closer to, or clearer about, what we choose to create. So the pattern of results looks something like this." She drew a squiggly line that seemed to trend upward.

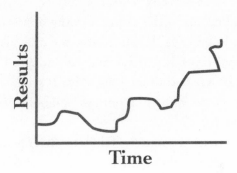

"Sometimes it is a step forward and other times it may be a step back, but over time you make progress toward your outcome."

I thought to myself, Hmm... while I thought I was simply on a roller coaster, my week was actually more like the second graph. That surprised me. I'd made some progress, took some steps back, but – on balance – I had to count the week as a positive.

It was such a relief to let go of the unrealistic expectation that I'd always be in forward motion. It wasn't always going to be "goodness and light" and a continuous series of breakthroughs. Rather, I would take a Baby Step at a time.

I leaned over to Ram and said, "Light bulb!"

Ram grinned.

Marianne said, "Time is almost up for tonight's session, so let me give you another homework assignment. Reflect on what health, well-being and vitality would look like in your life. What is your vision? I encourage you to journal about it, and perhaps discuss this with your friends and family. I'll see you at our next class!"

I walked up to the man from the alumni group before I left and said, "Hi, Mark, my name is Joe. I can see why you like this class. Adopting a Creator Orientation is definitely a big shift. It gives me a lot to think about in dealing with my diabetes. It really gives me hope."

He shook my hand. "Glad to meet you, Joe. Yeah, I know what you mean about this way of thinking – way of living, actually. The first time I heard Marianne present that Creator Orientation, I nearly came out of my chair. One of the major takeaways from this class was this orientation. I am really doing my best to practice this proactive mind-set and to make it my way of approaching all of my life – including creating health."

I nodded, "I'm not ready to say that I'm grateful for my diabetes," I told him as we walked into the parking lot, "But I am glad to have this new understanding of how this works. I don't want to get ahead of myself. I think applying it to my diabetes and creating health is enough for me right now. There are plenty of Baby Steps to do. That said, this is really, really helpful stuff."

"If you think this is helpful, just wait," Mark said. "The next class will build on what you heard today and totally shift your relationship to the disease and how to deal with it."

"Well, I'll be back. That's for sure!"

A Different Way of Relating

I was in the best of moods when I got home from class. The family was sprawled around the den watching TV. I slipped in beside Lois on the couch and gave her a quick peck on the cheek. She smiled "Well, good to see you too!"

I laughed, "We had a great class tonight. After the show I want to tell you all about it."

Lois stood up, "I've thought a lot about what we said last night." Taking my hand she said, "Hearing about your class is more important than watching this show. Let's go to the kitchen and you can tell me what you learned."

Using the handout from class, I excitedly explained the elements of the Creator Orientation. She listened intently. When I explained the difference between trying to get away from the problem and the accompanying anxiety compared to working toward a desired outcome, a bright smile spread across her face.

"Interesting! I can see how what we focus on can make a big difference. Is it really that simple and easy?" She cocked her head to the side in mock suspicion. "I sure hope this works."

"Yeah, me too." I was aware that a shift had happened in my thinking and approach and was looking forward to focusing on what I wanted, rather than trying somehow to get away from my diabetes.

In the following days, I felt like I couldn't be stopped. Instead of feeling victimized over what I couldn't eat, I made food choices based on which ones would support my overall health. Each night after work, I had plenty of energy to take my walk. In fact, I started jogging part of the way and played around with the idea of joining the lunch break jogging group at work. I started taking the stairs at work, instead of the elevator, to my third-floor office.

Each morning my numbers declined bit by bit. I was really delighted when my pants weren't quite a snug as usual. Guess I'm Baby Stepping along pretty well.

For the next week and a half, I applied the model, not just to my health, but to other aspects of my life as well. At work I caught myself a number of times reacting to a problem. I would then stop and ask myself, what is the outcome I want?

At home it seemed like a miracle solution to dealing with the kids. When they complained or re-sisted doing their homework, I asked them, "What outcome do you want?" Together we brainstormed possibilities. They seemed empowered by con-sciously thinking about their own choices. There just seemed to be less anger and drama.

This era of bliss came to a crashing end the weekend before the next class. I slept in late that Saturday morning and was still tired when I got up. Lois put a cup of coffee in front of me and said,

"We both got an email from your cousin asking about our plans to attend your family reunion next summer."

"Oh," I scowled. "I wish he'd stop bugging us about that."

Lois sat down next to me, "Well, Joe. If we're going to fly, we've got to make reservations sooner rather than later. Otherwise it will cost too much."

I said, "We can always drive."

Lois frowned at me. "You know I don't want to drive half way across the country! It would take us days. And having the kids in the backseat the entire way…No, Joe. If we go, we fly."

Before I could say anything, the kids came into the kitchen. JJ asked, "Fly where?"

Lois said, "To the family reunion."

Our daughter frowned and turned to Lois, "Ah, mom. Do we have to go?"

Lois leaned back in her chair, "Well, that's a question to ask your father."

I knew I had no choice. I had to go to the re-union or never hear the end of it from my extended family. I didn't want to tell everyone there about my diabetes. I still felt out of shape. I didn't think I could ever keep up with my cousin, Mr. I'm-In-Perfect-Shape, on the mountain hike he had planned. I sighed, "Yes, we all have to go."

The complaints continued. Lisa whined, "I don't want to go. I want to stay here and go to soccer camp, not hang around with a bunch of people I don't really know that well. They ask all kinds of annoying questions."

With a touch of heavy sarcasm my son declared, "The outcome I want is to stay home!"

I blew up, "That's enough! We're all going. Your mom and I will decide if we drive or fly. Staying home is out of the question." I got up and left the room before anything else could be said.

After that, I lost my momentum completely. Instead of working it out with Lois, I pulled away and retreated to the den to check email. When she wasn't looking, I snuck a cold piece of leftover pizza and a beer. This started a couple days of a downward spiral and an increase in my numbers.

CHAPTER

SIX

Making Shifts Happen

With mixed emotions, I walked into the next class. I was embarrassed by my back steps, but I also knew I needed more support than I was getting. It didn't take long to shake my blues, however. The regular attendees had gotten to know each other, so there were plenty of "hello's" and "how was your week?" greetings.

Laughter buoyed me up and I connected with some of the people I'd met over the past couple of months. I also noticed that there were more people than any previous class and several new faces. Ram and I sat next to each other as Marianne went to the front of the class. I was surprised to see several of the regulars from the alumni group slip in with smiles on their faces. "This must be another important class." I said to the Ram.

Marianne said, "Welcome to the fourth class of 'Empowered Living with Diabetes.' We have a strange track record with this week's class – it always seems to be the most attended. Many graduates of the series come back for a review session. How many fall into that category tonight?" About a quarter of the hands went up.

"This is the class where the pieces of what we have been exploring come together. I predict that, after this class, you will not only have the basis for a new relationship with your diabetes, but also a new relationship framework for how you engage with your doctors and the healthcare system, as well as a whole new way of relating to family, friends, and the rest of your life experience."

I leaned over to Ram, "And not a moment too soon."

Marianne continued, "As you make the shift from a problem-focused, anxiety or fear-fueled and reactive Victim Orientation to a more empowered and resourceful Creator Orientation, a much different set of relationship roles and dynamics become possible. Rather than engaging in the toxic brew of the Victim, Persecutor, and Rescuer roles in the Dreaded Drama Triangle, we can now cultivate The Empowerment Dynamic." She wrote *TED** and an upward-facing triangle on the whiteboard.

TED*

"The three roles we are going to explore serve as the antidote to the toxic DDT roles. We're going to take them one at a time. Before we do, however, I want to acknowledge that the framework we are about to explore comes from the inspiring insights of Dr. Theresa Elizabeth Davis – or Dr. Ted as those of us who know her like to call her."

"Yea, Dr. Ted!" a man called out from the back of the room and the room broke out in laughter.

Marianne smiled "Thank you for that appreciative acknowledgement."

For the next hour, Marianne explained TED* to us, and I could see that I needed to sit down with Lois and go over this material with her. I got an extra set of handouts and headed home with renewed determination to pursue the life I wanted to achieve, rather than spiral back into reactive, fear-based behavior.

Armed with my handouts, and a combination of courage and humility, I headed home to talk with Lois. As usual, I found her in the family room with the kids watching TV.

"Lois?" I asked, to get her attention.

She turned her face toward me.

"Can we take a few minutes and discuss what I learned tonight?"

She sighed. She had grown weary of my radical swings between high-energy optimism and irritability. With a half smile she said, "Well, since I'm not going to divorce you…yet…I guess I have no other choice."

"Yet?"

She poked me in the arm. "That was a joke, Joe." I decided not to dwell on her comment. We walked into the kitchen and sat at our table.

I handed her a set of the handouts, and then looked down at my own. "Lois, I want to go over what we discussed in the class tonight. I think it's really important, not only to my health, but to our relationship, and for our family."

She stopped me. "OK, Joe. But I need to say that while I appreciate you including me, I just hope it makes a difference for you, me, and all of us. I feel like I've been going through emotional whiplash. You go to class and come back enthused and then drop into crankiness and despair. It's gotten old. "

"I know, honey. It's been very hard on you and the kids."

She patted my hand. "I don't want to be a discouragement to you. So, OK, tell me what you learned tonight."

Feeling somewhat more affirmed by her, I launched in and pointed to the page that showed the DDT and TED* triangles side by side. "Do you remember the Dreaded Drama Triangle?"

"Oh, yes." She replied.

"Well, tonight we learned about TED* (*The Empowerment Dynamic). As you can see, this triangle is the flip side of the DDT triangle. It's pointed up instead of down, and is what Marianne called the antidote to the toxic roles described in the DDT. The role of Victim, which is at the bottom of

the DDT triangle, is replaced by the *Creator* role."
On the side of the diagram I pointed to "Creator."

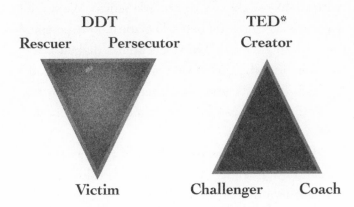

DDT

Rescuer   Persecutor

Victim

TED*

Creator

Challenger   Coach

"Hmm." Lois said, "I sure like the idea of being creative better than victimized."

I nodded. "Me too. There are two primary characteristics of being a Creator. The first is that we focus on the outcomes we care about – like health and well-being."

Lois teased, "Or envisioning the possibility of missing the family reunion?"

I chuckled, "Well, that would be focusing on what we don't want. Maybe we can focus on a fun family reunion. " I looked back at the handouts to remember the second Creator characteristic.

I said, "The second part is just as important. As a Creator, we can choose our response to the situations that arise in our lives – even when we feel victimized by other people or situations – like being diagnosed with diabetes. The mantra of a Creator is to 'Choose Choice'."

Lois nodded as she took this in. I leaned back in my chair. "Everyone at the class has been diagnosed with diabetes. But we're not 'diabetics'. We are all Creators who have diabetes." I made it more personal by declaring. "I am a Creator who has diabetes."

Lois added, "So how you respond to your diagnosis depends upon whether you react to it as a Victim or choose how to respond as a Creator, right?"

"Exactly. Marianne continually tells us that, as Creators, we can live happy, healthy, fulfilling lives – even with diabetes. But if we assume the role of Victim, we spend our time reacting to our diagnosis as a problem or Persecutor. As a Creator, I can respond to diabetes as a *Challenger*, which is the antidote to the DDT role of Persecutor." On the handout, I circled the word "Challenger."

"When a Challenger shows up in our life, whether as a person, circumstance or a condition like diabetes, it provides an opportunity to learn and grow. The Challenger is a teacher to a Creator. A Challenger evokes or provokes a call to action. As a Creator, I ask, 'What has this Challenger come into my life to cause me to learn, grow, or develop in response?'"

Lois said, "That's a lot more helpful than asking, 'Why me?'"

"Yes," I agreed.

"And you know what, Joe? Even though your diabetes has been so difficult for you, for all of us, it's bringing this new information into our lives that will help all of us in our family make positive changes. I guess I'm grateful for that part."

I added, "Marianne told us that everyone, not just those of us with diabetes, has Challengers in life. We all have unwelcome and unwanted events, circumstances...even people. Unconscious Challengers are anyone or anything that challenge us even when they are not aware that they are doing so."

"Like the kids," Lois laughed.

"That's for sure!" I laughed with her.

The Need for a Challenger

"There is another, more positive kind of Challenger that can be very important and very helpful that Marianne described. It is a person who is acting as a 'Conscious Constructive Challenger' and who sees you as a Creator. They challenge, cajole, or nudge you in support of your learning, growth, and development."

"I think that's what I've wanted to be," Lois admitted.

I said, "Yes. I think you have. And I think my former doctor wanted to do that too. Even though some of us in the class had trouble seeing some of the health care providers in a positive light, Marianne insists that our doctors and others in the medical field really do want us to learn how to manage our diabetes.

"She pointed out that, unfortunately, many in the healthcare system are less-than-conscious Challengers in the way they push us to exercise, watch what we eat, lose weight, and stuff. I'll admit that she's probably right. Their intentions are good. She said she was encouraged that there are more and more doctors, diabetes educators, and others who are challenging in conscious and constructive ways."

"The third part of the triangle in TED* is the role of *Coach*. As a Creator, I need support from the Coaches in my life." I pointed to "Coach" on the page. This is the antidote to the DDT role of Rescuer. A Coach sees you as a Creator, whether you know it or not, or are acting like it or not.

"In the DDT, even though Rescuers are trying to be helpful, since they see us as Victims, they un-intentionally reinforce our sense of powerlessness. Coaches, on the other hand, see us as Creators and as being ultimately capable and resourceful. Instead of telling us what to do or how to fix our problems, they ask questions that help us clarify our outcomes and to decide how to respond to life's challenges."

"When Marianne was explaining the Coach role, I recalled how Dr. Ted coached me about how I could remind myself to take my medication in the evening, rather than giving me suggestions or telling me how to do it.

"So there you have it. TED* (*The Empowerment

Dynamic) and its three roles of Creator, Challenger, and Coach. Pretty good stuff, don't you think?"

Lois responded, "What an amazing difference all of this could make!"

We both sat in silence as we thought about the implications of TED* for our own lives. Lois spoke up first, "I've wanted to help you, but haven't really known how. I can see how my attempts have been based on the fear that you weren't really capable of dealing with this. I think I have been alternating between wanting to be a Rescuer and then being a bit of a Persecutor." She stroked my arm. "I have doubted you, and you picked up on that."

I put my hand over hers, "Lois, you were half right. Even though I am capable of creating a healthy life, not playing the Victim to diabetes, I didn't have the tools to be successful until now. I feel like I have a whole new set of tools and skills I didn't have just a few short months ago. Most importantly, I have a whole new way of thinking and approaching life. I know this is going to take a lot of work, but I think I... I mean, I think we can do this."

She kissed me on the forehead. "You're right, Joe. We all have a new way of looking at all of the curves life throws us from a much more empowered mind-set. You and I will have to put our heads together and find a way that engages all of us, even the kids, that empowers us to deal with the DFR."

"DFR?" I asked, perplexed.

"The Dreaded Family Reunion!"

It was good to laugh with Lois again. With us working from the same page (sometimes literally), the next two weeks were the most enjoyable I'd had since receiving my diagnosis. Sure, there were days when I nibbled on snacks that pushed up my numbers, or days when I opted to hang out with my buddies to watch football all Sunday afternoon and didn't get any exercise for myself. But all in all, I was more of a Creator than a Victim, and I treated myself with more kindness when I messed up than I had before.

I also felt good about how I interacted with my children, at least for the most part. There was one Saturday afternoon when my son popped two frozen burritos into the oven. I asked, "Are you going to eat both of them?"

"Sure, why not?" he asked.

"Well, they are full of sodium and fat and..."

"Dad." He gave me one of his bothered looks. "Well, at least they are vegetarian. Isn't that what you and Lisa are into these days? So, can you get off your high horse? Just because you're old and sickly doesn't mean I am."

I felt like he punched me in the stomach. "It's not about being old and I am not sick! I developed diabetes because I wasn't aware of all the little things that added up after years and years. Plus, the tendency to develop diabetes runs in our family. I'm just trying to protect you."

"Please *stop*! I can protect myself." he said, grabbing the burritos from the oven. "I'm going over to Carl's house. At least over there I don't have to have the food police breathing down my neck."

Lois walked into the kitchen as he stomped out.

I gave her a sad smile, "Well, that went well."

"It's okay, Joe. He's at that age where he wants to start being viewed as a young adult and probably is frustrated with all the changes we're going through as a family to cope with your diabetes."

I sighed, "I know. Trust me, I wish I never developed diabetes. Some days I try to ignore it, but soon my numbers go up, and I feel scared. There is no going back. As someone joked in class, De-Nile is more than a river in Egypt. As corny as the joke was, I know denial is a dangerous place to go. I swear it will get better before long. At least I hope so."

The Commitment Behind the Complaint

Before I knew it, it was time for the next class. Since it seemed like we'd already learned the key concepts that were working, I wondered what else Marianne had up her sleeve.

I walked into the class and saw written on the whiteboard "Making Shifts Happen." Below the words was a large six-pointed asterisk with both the DDT and TED* roles:

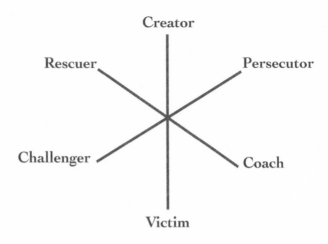

Creator

Rescuer

Persecutor

Challenger

Coach

Victim

Marianne welcomed everyone and then said, "Who says the medical profession doesn't have a sense of humor? Today we are going to address a very important topic, even though the title is a little corny. You may have noticed since last class that it is so, so easy to slip back into the drama roles.

"Why is it so easy to slip, you might ask? Because we are human and the Victim Orientation and the Dreaded Drama Triangle are our default way of operating as human beings. What we are really putting into place in this class is a new Personal Operating Mind-set – you could call it a POM Pilot," she said with a wry smile. "Get it?"

A chuckle slowly emerged from the class. "This operating system will be useful in every facet of your life, including how you relate to and can meet the challenge of your diabetes.

"When we find ourselves in one of the drama roles, it is important to know how to escape the drama and get back into TED*. So let's explore how we can make shifts happen."

She passed out a handout and then pointed to the whiteboard. "The first shift is the core shift – from Victim to Creator. As we talked about several classes ago, the primary questions to ask are 'what do I want?' and 'how do I choose to respond?' This may be easier said than done, however."

"Have you been following me around?" a man on the front row asked. "I said to a friend at work yesterday that this stuff seems simple, but that it's certainly not easy." I suspected we all felt that way. All through this course, Marianne seemed to be able to describe exactly what I'd been thinking and feeling.

"You are so right," she responded, "it *is* simple, but not easy. The place to begin is to ask yourself the core questions of what you want and how you choose to respond. In thinking about what you want, you will see on the handout that I have added a few other questions that can lead to powerful answers."

I looked at the sheet and was actually inspired by the questions:

* What am I committed to?
* What future do I see is possible for me, and for my family?
* What is possible for me to achieve?

As if out of the blue, I had an 'aha' moment! I felt a tear well in my eye.

I glanced around hoping no one would notice. But to myself, I said with conviction softly and aloud, "I will not yield to diabetes, I will see my grandchildren graduate from high school with my eyes, feet, and kidneys operating normally. I will overcome this challenge!"

I knew something fundamental had changed in me—a shift in the foundation of my life perspective. It felt almost spiritual. Even if no one around me could tell the difference in me, I knew. I knew.

I tuned back in to what Marianne was saying. "Sometimes the answers to these questions come quickly. Other times we may need to look more deeply at what we are experiencing that we don't like for clues about what we really want.

"First, any time we are in the Victim role it is because there is some dream or desire that is being denied or thwarted.

"Second, if we find ourselves complaining, then I can guarantee we are being a Victim. Think about it. If we didn't care about something, we wouldn't be complaining. So identifying what it is you care about or what the dream or desire is that you want becomes the key to making this shift happen.

"Let me ask you--What dream or desire is being denied or thwarted by your diabetes?"

A number of people answered:

"Being able to eat whatever I want."

"Feeling normal."

"Being healthy."

"Letting my kids have a normal childhood," I said.

Marianne affirmed our answers, "Good, the commitments behind the complaints and the dreams denied are health and a fulfilling everyday life. Receiving the diagnosis of diabetes is a 'wake-up call' to health and well being, which requires conscious focus and effort. While there is no going back to sleep and resuming our old unhealthy ways – at least in the long run – if you want to create a long, healthy, and fulfilling life, you *can* move forward in empowered ways as a Creator.

"The essence of this shift is *moving from reacting to choosing*. Choosing health and wellbeing, as well as choosing how to respond to the realities of diabetes, is what this shift is all about.

"As a Creator with diabetes, I also encourage you to become a fearless activated patient in working with your healthcare support system. Be proactive with your doctor. All of us – patients, doctors, and healthcare providers – need to move from our drama roles and relate to one another as Creators. This is about health empowerment."

Marianne looked around the room. "I want to ask you all a tough question. Has it been hard to ask for help through this process?"

Several people nodded. I raised my hand, "It was embarrassing to admit I had diabetes at all. I even resisted taking medication for a while. Asking for help seemed too much to bear."

Marianne nodded in understanding. "There is no weakness in seeking support and help. As a Creator, you retain the responsibility for making the choices and taking the Baby Steps that will lead to a new lifestyle and life. Rather than seeing me, or your doctor, or others as Rescuers who are going to somehow fix it and make it all better, utilize them as a Coach to support you in making informed choices.

"For those of you who can, you might consider finding a health coach – there are more and more practitioners joining the field every day. One of the newer trends with health insurance companies is that they are beginning to provide or cover the cost of health coaching and health education across the United States. Sadly the biggest problem with these programs is the lack of willingness of people with diabetes to work with them and participate. Don't let that be you!

"That said, the Coach role in TED* does not have to be a professional coach. One of the things I love about the alumni group, that you are invited to attend after you complete this class, is how participants serve one another through coaching.

"The primary contribution of a Coach is to ask questions that help a Creator clarify their envisioned outcomes and to see alternative ways or choices that they can make in response to the challenges they face. They also help others identify and commit to the next Baby Step that will help them move forward.

"Lastly, let's talk about the Persecutor to Challenger shift. We've already talked about how diabetes itself is a Challenger that is sparking learning, growth, and development in your lives every day. Your choosing to be in this class is an indicator that you are making shift happen away from reacting to it as a Persecutor to choosing to see it as a Challenger . With time you may actually come to see your diabetes as a gift – I know I have."

Marianne instructed us to pull out our handout. "On this sheet, there's an exercise I'd like you all to do right now. You'll see a list of seven blank lines. I want you to list seven ways in which diabetes has been a teacher or a gift to you. You may not get all the way through the list tonight, but I want you to get a good start."

I thought to myself, there's no way I could have filled this out just a few weeks ago. Now I see things a bit differently. I started my list with:

1. Learning about food so I can make healthier choices about what I eat
2. Starting to lose weight (something I seem to have always struggled with)
3. Feeling better than I have in a long time
4. Learning how my body works, i.e. what the pancreas does

After a few minutes of silence, Marianne said to us, "There are times when your healthcare providers need to serve as a supporting Challenger to you. When they do, it is important to remember that they are serving you by encouraging you to grow through learning about your diabetes and how to effectively manage it for yourself.

"At times, I have also seen alumni group members step up to being a conscious, constructive Challenger. The key to being a constructive Challenger to others is to be clear about the intent behind your challenging. There is an important distinction between challenging from a 'looking good intent' versus a 'learning intent' from which we share and teach others. If you challenge someone in order to look good – to be right, to be a hero/fixer, in other words, a Rescuer, to show you are smarter than or better than the other, how do you think they are going to respond to you? Will they perceive you as a Persecutor or a Challenger?"

I spoke up, "That's easy! They will react to you as a Persecutor."

Marianne nodded. "It's virtually guaranteed. Conscious, constructive Challengers challenge from a learning intention. First and foremost, they view the person they are challenging as a Creator in their own right – whether they know it or not, or act like it or not. Remember, Challengers spark learning and growth."

I reflected back on my conversation with JJ about his burrito. I had to admit part of me was trying to teach him, but part of me was trying to tell him what to do. Even though I was trying to help, he clearly reacted to me as a Persecutor.

Marianne pulled me out of my thoughts. "See the asterisk in TED*? Have you wondered why I always include that? It represents the fact that we are always at choice, and have the capacity to shift from the roles of the Dreaded Drama Triangle to those of The Empowerment Dynamic. It's a 'choice point'," she emphasized as she pointed to the asterisk on the whiteboard.

I left the class committed to making conscious choices. This wasn't just about my diabetes – it was about my quality of life and my relationship with my family.

CHAPTER

SEVEN

Harnessing Dynamic Tension

The next two weeks, we all did well as a family and I did a great job with my diabetes management. The kids grew more comfortable with the changes as we learned to use the ways of thinking and relating to one another that I had gained from the class.

We served as coaches for one another in a way that actually helped, rather than annoyed, each of us. My becoming more active, settling into a new way of eating, and tracking progress with my numbers were becoming routine – almost.

I was sailing along until Saturday night when Lois took the kids to a movie. I'd had a long week at work and opted to stay home on my own to rest and reflect over the past week.

Or at least that was what I intended to do. As I was rooting around through the kitchen drawers for a pen to write in my journal, I opened the snack drawer and found a half-eaten bag of potato chips. Ah…the bag wasn't sealed and I could smell the wonderful aroma of grease and potatoes.

I realized that no one was around to catch me in the act and before I could get a grip on myself, I had plopped down on the sofa in the family room with the remote in my hand. I sprawled out, mindlessly watched TV, and devoured the rest of the bag.

Man, did I enjoy the taste of the salt and seasonings! It had been a long time since I'd savored that taste. After all, I deserved this! I had been doing so well, how could a few potato chips hurt? Already on a roll, I looked through the cupboards and found a box of cookies — my favorite kind. By the time my family returned, the empty bags were hidden outside in the bottom of the trash can. I acted like I'd just pulled off the perfect crime. If only it were that easy.

The next morning my blood sugar told the truth. Lois happened to see the meter and raised an eyebrow at me. I gave no explanation. I knew exactly what had happened, and I wasn't in the mood to deal with her disappointment in my behavior. I went to class that week with my tail between my legs.

Marianne called us to order and said, "Welcome to the next-to-last class, folks! Did I tell you that there would be a test tonight?"

There was an audible gasp in the room. Voices spoke up, "What?" "No!" "You gotta be kidding!"

Marianne laughed, "I guess no one likes tests in here!" A few of us chuckled at ourselves. She continued, "Well, yes, I am kidding – sort of. We will get to the mini-test in a minute. First I want to do a quick review.

"Over the past few months we have talked about SARAH, FISBE, the Dreaded Drama Triangle (DDT), the Victim and Creator Orientations, TED* (*The Empowerment Dynamic), and how we make shifts happen. The final major framework that I want to share with you tonight is called Dynamic Tension.[1] It is a very simple way of planning for and taking action to create outcomes, and to stay more consistently in a Creator Orientation. I call it the 3-step dance of creating.

"First, here's the test. Are you ready? It is one question: If you choose to live from a Creator Orientation, where do you put your focus? Remember FISBE – Focus, Inner State, and Behavior? What is the focus of a Creator?"

"Outcomes."

"Vision."

"Choice."

"Great – you all pass with flying colors!"

She wrote *Vision/Outcome* at the top of the whiteboard. "In creating outcomes you always start by focusing on what you want to create. You start by answering the question, 'What do I want?'

---

1   Dynamic Tension is derived from Robert Fritz's brilliant description of the creative process, most notably in his books *The Path of Least Resistance* and *Creating*.

"The second question comes from Robert Fritz's work with what he calls 'structural tension.' It is an important and powerful question to ask yourself, 'If I had what I want, how would I know it?' This forces you to identify the qualities, characteristics or other components of the envisioned outcome.

"A couple of classes ago, I gave you homework to reflect on what well-being, health, and vitality would look like for you. If you had optimal health and well-being, how would you know it?"

A man in the front said, "I'd have more energy."

"People would say I look good," said a woman next to him.

A woman to my left said, "My diabetes would be under control."

I spoke up, as in confession, "I'd be eating healthy food."

Ram said, "I'd lose weight."

Marianne said, "Ah…I don't want to pick on you, Ram, but I want to use your comment as a way to illustrate a point. It's really important to set your intentions and envision outcomes in affirmative language. Focus on what you want, rather than what you don't want. The words 'lose weight' places your energy on what you want to get rid of. It is subtle, I know, but what is a more affirmative statement you could make about your weight?"

Ram thought for a moment, and then said, "I would be able to wear some of my old, favorite clothes."

"Good, you see yourself wearing old – and maybe some new – smaller clothes."

The woman to my left chimed in: "I'd like what I see in the mirror!"

Marianne nodded. "Do you see how those statements are more powerful – and empowering – than merely seeing it as losing weight? How would it feel to say, 'I am at my preferred body weight?'"

There were nods all around the room.

Marianne explained, "Merely envisioning the outcome and identifying how you would know it if you had it is not sufficient for creating it. Intention alone does not bring the vision or outcome into being.

"The second step in the process is assessing your current reality in relation to the outcome." She wrote *Current Reality* about half-way down the whiteboard right below *Vision/Outcome* and drew a line connecting them.

"In order to move toward your vision you need to know where you currently are. If I were to take you out to some remote location, drop you off and then say 'I'll meet you back here,' you'd have to know where you were – what your current reality was – so that you knew in what direction to begin walking. Assessing current reality must be made honestly and accurately if you want to succeed."

Definitely a Stretch

Marianne reached into her briefcase and pulled out a bag of rubber bands. She took one out and handed the bag to the person sitting in front of her. "Please take a rubber band and pass the bag to the next person."

While the bag made its way around the room, she continued. "By identifying your intended outcome and assessing current reality, you engage a force – a tension – between the two that is best illustrated by the rubber band you have in your hand.

"Take the rubber band and put it over your two index fingers. One finger represents your outcome and the other your current reality. Now stretch them apart. "Do you feel the tension?"

We all did.

"If the rubber band could talk, what would it say it wants to do right now?"

Various people spoke up. "Relax!"

"Come together."

"Contract."

"Yes," Marianne agreed, "It is a structure that seeks resolution. We call it Dynamic Tension. It's an important component of TED*. It is a dynamic, creative experience which is always in play as we create and co-create with others."

I raised my hand, "Are you saying that I'm going to live in this kind of tension for the rest of my life? Even though you have consistently told us that you aren't going to save us, I keep waiting to land some-where that is no longer difficult. I'm tired of trying so hard, only to fall short of my goal. I want my life to be as easy as it was before my diagnosis."

Marianne smiled, "Honestly, folks. I didn't ask him to say this, but Joe, your comment is the perfect bridge over to the next point I want to make. Your life may have seemed easier before your diagnosis because it was so familiar to you, but let me ask you something: were you proactive in your life or reactive?"

I smiled, "I was reactive all the way."

"And which Orientation did that put you into?"

"Victim," I responded.

"And what is the inner experience of being in the Victim Orientation?"

I knew the answer to that. "Anxiety."

Marianne continued, "So what you describe as being an easier way of life was actually one filled with anxiety as you reacted to whatever came your way."

I mulled that over for a moment. "Yes, I see that now. It seemed easier because I didn't have to think about what I wanted or what I was going to do. I just reacted to my situation and tried to push down the anxiety I felt."

"That's right. Since you didn't identify what you wanted out of life or set any goals – especially as it concerned your health - you never put effort into reaching those goals."

I smiled, "Great. I had no direction and was plagued with fear. Well, that doesn't sound so easy."

Marianne looked out at the class. "Do any of you identify with Joe?"

Hands shot up all over the room. Someone in the back of the room said, "Oh, give me the good old days of wandering aimlessly filled with terror!"

The class laughed. Marianne said, "It's easy to romanticize how we all lived before our diagnosis woke us up from living an unexamined existence. You might say we were sleepwalking though life. And, yes, being in that Victim role of just reacting to whatever comes up in life may seem easier because it's familiar. In reality, being a Victim isn't easy at all. It takes a great deal of effort."

What an insight into the way I used to live my life! I had no idea that I had been so out of control in the way I was living. Just because it was familiar, doesn't mean it was actually easier or beneficial.

Marianne interrupted my musings when she asked, "Are we ready to get back to our rubber bands?"

We put the bands around our index fingers. I had to laugh. "We are so trainable," I whispered to Ram.

She continued, "We've seen that we can't avoid stress in our lives, no matter what role we play. Tension is inherent in being alive. So, I suggest we make the most of it."

Someone close to the front said, "Here! Here!"

Marianne said, "When you engage this tension between what you want, which is your vision, and where you are, which is your current reality, you can expect to experience some sort of anxiety about the road ahead of you.

"Now I'm going to say something important that may be a bit of a disappointment initially -- anxiety comes with the territory of being a Creator. It's easy for this feeling to pull us back into the Victim role. If we do not stay aware and diligent, the anxiety we feel in the process of creating can very easily pull us back into the Victim Orientation where we will react to the fear."

I spoke up again. "Wait a minute, Marianne. Are you saying that we will feel anxiety whether we are in the Victim or Creator roles?"

Marianne affirmed. "Yes, actually. Being a Creator is not anxiety-free."

A groan could be heard around the room. Marianne smiled, but continued, "As we've discussed, you may automatically react to anxiety by reverting to the Victim perspective. As a Creator you develop a much more resourceful way of dealing with anxiety. The more you live your life as a Creator, the more you will learn to respond – rather than just react – to the anxiety. Part of being a Creator is being able to move forward even in the face of the anxiety you are feeling.

"However, if we fall back into the Victim Orientation, there are two ways to resolve the tension between our vision and current reality, both of which are really reactions intended to make the anxiety go away."

Marianne stretched out the rubber band between her hands. "Remember which hand represents your envisioned outcome and which one current reality. What is the easiest way to react that will lessen the tension."

Ram said, "Move my hands closer together."

"Yes, but, if you could only move one hand, which one would be the easiest to alter – your vision or your current reality?"

Ram looked a bit perplexed, and eventually, more asked than stated, "It would be easiest to alter my vision?"

She responded. "So you could compromise your vision by moving your vision finger toward your current reality." Marianne moved her vision hand closer to the one representing the current reality. "See how the tension gets released? By doing this, we give up what we really want."

I thought about my chips and cookies binge. I had released a lot of anxiety by eating, but by the next morning, I was struggling under a burden of even more intense shame and fear. My choices had clearly moved me further away from my vision of healthy eating, although the experience of giving up my goal was temporarily satisfying.

Marianne continued, "There is a second way we can react to the anxiety that is not helpful in the long run. Instead of compromising the vision, we could react by not telling the truth about our current reality. We can deny, rationalize and/or minimize where we are and what we are doing. I don't know about you, but I can tell you that it was months and months – actually the better part of a year – before I accepted and really looked at the current reality of my diabetes when I was first diagnosed."

I knew exactly what Marianne was talking about. I thought, I guess I should be glad that it only took me a few months to face it.

Marianne looked around the group, "None of us wants to be known as a liar. Most of us value honesty and truth-telling. Yet being honest with ourselves can be a big challenge when we don't want to face what is real.

"Now that you are better equipped to deal with the truth, it can be significantly easier to acknowledge the current reality. In the past, acknowledging your diagnosis added tension and anxiety to your life, pulling you further into a Victim response. But that's not your only alternative now."

Harnessing the Tension

"Here's the way to really harness and to tap into this Dynamic Tension to create your envisioned outcomes." She rather dramatically moved her current reality hand closer to the hand that represented her envisioned future. "If you hold to your vision *and* you tell the truth about your current reality, you achieve what you want by taking action to move *from* your current reality *toward* your vision as you embrace the Creator perspective. Anticipate anxiety—and learn to dance with it.

"Don't rush to relieve it, or see it as 'bad.' Learn to acknowledge it as uncomfortable, but healthy. It is the energy that is moving you toward the most important goals in your life. I've heard it said that 'dissatisfaction breeds change,' well in this case the dissatisfaction breeds your personal success. Over time you may actually convert it into excitement in the process of creating. Again, it is important to know that being a Creator is not anxiety-free."

A man in the front held up his hand. Marianne nodded in his direction. He said, "I don't know if this is the time to ask this question, but I have had no support from my wife through this process. I have invited her to class, but she won't come. The more I share the TED* concepts with her, the more annoyed she seems to be. Is there a way I can get my wife on board with dealing with my diabetes?"

Marianne thought for a moment. "Let's step back from this a moment and look at the bigger picture. Applying these principles to your life changes the way you live your life in total—it's not just about managing your diabetes. If all any of us had to do was take a pill, then none of us would be here in this class tonight. The fact that diabetes confronts us with the way we live, not merely how we cope with illness, causes a significant wave of change. When we change, our friends and family are confronted with change as well."

The man nodded his head. "Yes, that's true. At first, I felt so victimized by all of this. Now, I'm actually energized by the larger ramifications. I feel so alive these days. My wife, on the other hand, longs for me to go back to being the man I used to be. It's been very hard on our marriage."

Marianne said, "There's no easy answer for me to give you. As you envision a deeper, more conscious relationship with your wife, and work toward that, she may choose to join you in the growth process. Sometimes spouses don't make that choice."

Silence settled over the group as we each thought about the impact our diabetes, and now our empowered response, was having on our families and friends. I thought to myself, I am so grateful that Lois has hung in with me, and is actually embracing the changes as positive. When I get home tonight, I'm going to let her know how much I appreciate her.

Marianne broke the silence by saying, "I don't want to end on a depressing note. I hope that all of you will move forward, and not succumb to the anxiety by retreating back to a Victim role."

Heads nodded in agreement. "Two weeks from tonight is the last session in the series. We will focus on identifying and taking Baby Steps, small actions that take us closer and closer toward our envisioned lives."

I turned to Ram once the class ended and said, "Well, it looks like no matter which way we go, we have to learn how to deal with anxiety—either caused by being a Victim or as a by-product of intentionally going for our envisioned outcome."

Ram smiled, and said sarcastically, "Yes. And on top of that, we are challenged by those in our lives who are impacted by our choices. Now isn't that good news?"

We both chuckled. "For me, it makes anxiety seem much less ferocious. So what if there's some anxiety in my life? I don't have to operate under the illusion that if I get it right, I'll always feel on top of the world."

Ram agreed. "It definitely takes the pressure off." As we walked to our cars he said, "Well, our last class is coming up. When I first heard about this class I thought, 'Oh, no - six classes! That's too long,' but it's gone so fast."

"Yes," I responded, "it's gone more quickly than I expected too. I like the idea of the alumni group. I think I'll go to that, I need all the support I can get. I think I'm in it for the long haul."

CHAPTER

EIGHT

Taking Baby Steps

I was surprised to realize that it had been two months since I'd first visited Dr. Ted. While in the waiting room, I thought back on all I'd learned from Marianne in the class. I now approached Dr. Ted as a Coach and Challenger who would work with me as I took responsibility for creating health and well-being in my life.

Carson popped his head into the waiting room and called my name. It was good to see him again. He led me into an examination room and I noticed a chart on the wall that was very similar to the Dynamic Tension model that Marianne shared in the class. The caption over it read: "Supporting you in Creating a Healthy Life – A Baby Step at a Time."

I said, "I don't remember seeing that chart the last time I was in."

Carson said, "Very observant. When patients come to us for the first time, we take them to the exam room with the Creator Orientation diagram so that Dr. Ted can explain it. All of our other exam rooms have the Dynamic Tension chart in them."

Carson asked if there was anything to update on my record. My first impulse was to tell him how different my life was – my wife, kids, and I – how we were getting along, how we were grocery shopping differently, eating differently, doing more activities together; how I was getting more sleep, exercising at least 30 minutes five days a week, and how my blood sugars were consistently below 100 in the morning and 140 after meals. But I decided to save him the monologue – and the half-truth. All I said was, "Things are going pretty well."

He took my blood pressure, which was at the high end of the normal range, and was actually an improvement from months before. He then pointed to the scale for me to weigh in.

I was pleased to see that the scale confirmed what I already knew.

"You weigh 6 pounds less than last time." Carson congratulated me.

I beamed like a school boy finding a big 'A' on the top of his paper. I smiled in spite of myself.

Carson said as he left, "Marianne will be in shortly."

Marianne came in next and we talked about the improvements I had been making. Then she asked, "What do you want to accomplish in your session with Dr. Ted, Joe? What is the outcome that you want?"

I thought for a minute. "I want her to see the progress I have made. The other thing is for me to gain a better understanding of how to really manage my life with diabetes for the long haul."

She responded, "Perfect timing. That is what this appointment is really all about. Dr. Ted is with another patient, but you are up next. She will only be a few minutes."

I was left to my thoughts. I noticed how safe I felt in Dr. Ted's office. I was always so stressed with my previous doctor. Here I didn't feel criticized or put on the hot seat.

In a few minutes, Dr. Ted came in. Shaking my hand, she asked how I had been feeling.

I said, "Better, thanks. But I feel like I have just begun."

"That's a good perspective, Joe. You are very, very early in what is really a lifelong journey of growing into and maintaining optimal health. Let me take a few minutes to explain the format we will be using as we work together going forward."

I found it affirming that she believed I had a long lifetime ahead of me.

Dr. Ted looked at my chart and confirmed that I had continued to attend Marianne's class, so she said, "Since you are in the class, I don't need to re-explain the basic steps in Dynamic Tension. But I do want to emphasize that my role as your doctor is to support you as a Coach and, when necessary, as a Challenger – although I realize that diabetes is really your current primary Challenger."

I nodded in understanding.

"Let's work a little with Dynamic Tension," Dr. Ted said, "Joe, if you had health and well-being in your life, how would you know it?"

I answered with some of the same responses that arose in the last class: my numbers would be good; I would be wearing smaller size clothes because my weight would be lower...

Dr. Ted nodded as I rattled off the list, "Now, imagine for a minute that it is now next summer. What are you able to do now – again, it is next summer – which you could not do when you met with me last fall?"

I gave her a quizzical look. She said, "I know this is a bit artificial, because it is now fall, but play along with me."

"Okay," I agreed. I thought for a minute and then it hit me. "It's interesting that you should have me imagine it is next summer. I am going to be attending a big three-day family reunion. My cousin who is organizing it is a bit of a health nut, and he has issued a challenge to all of us of our generation to a 10-mile mountain hike the second day.

"It has been scary for me to consider it because I have been so out of shape. So, in my vision of next summer I see myself as healthy, in good shape, and able to do the hike without huffing and puffing the whole way."

She asked, "So you see yourself being able to successfully go on a ten-mile mountain hike in about nine months?"

"That would be awesome! Yes, that is my vision."

She smiled, "Great – that is what we will put out there for now as your vision of optimal health. What you will find, Joe, as you continue down this life-long path (no pun intended) is that as you achieve one vision – or one plateau – you will then set your sights on what's next, while taking the time to celebrate the achievement of each major milestone. That's another reason why we call this Dynamic Tension, because it is a driving force that is always changing and challenging us to higher effectiveness.

"Now we're going to look at your current reality. Your current state is where you find yourself at this time – not where you are going to stay. But before we do, I want to re-emphasize something I said during your first visit, and that is how important it is that you always be completely honest with me about your current state during checkups. I need you to accurately describe both what you are doing that supports your forward progress and where you might be struggling, falling back into the thinking or habits that lead to your situation when we met. For us to help you we must know the good, the bad, and the ugly of current reality. Can I rely on you to do that, Joe?"

"Message received loud and clear, Doc."

She looked at my chart and noted that my blood pressure had improved and that I'd lost six pounds since my first visit. She asked, "To what do you attribute the improvement?"

I listed off a number of changes I'd made—"My choice of foods with more protein, less refined and simple carbohydrates makes a big difference on how much I stress my pancreas and how much insulin my body has to produce.

"I'm improving my muscle uptake of blood sugar by walking five to six days a week, which has increased from thirty minutes to forty-five minutes or more each day. I am even jogging a little during the walks."

Dr. Ted smiled broadly and gently interrupted, "Gee, I can tell you have been learning more about what is going on in your body, Joe. You said that like a real seasoned veteran."

"Thanks, I am learning a lot. So is Lois, my wife. She walks with me most of the time, and now she's feeling and looking healthier. We've found a nearby park that has a 3-mile loop. At about the halfway point, there is a bench that looks out over a lake and hills. Just last week we were sitting there and Lois commented on how glad she is that we have taken responsibility for our health. We probably would never have found that bench if all this hadn't happened."

"That's a really good insight Lois had," Dr. Ted commented.

I am also careful to get 7-8 hours of sleep every night, and I am using breathing and relaxation techniques to handle stress more effectively. I'm surprised at how this seems to really help my blood sugar."

Dr. Ted said, "That's great, Joe, really great! Let's look at your lab report. Your fasting blood sugar is down thirty points from what it was when I met you. That's tremendous and your A1c is down almost a full point – that is as much as we could have hoped for. Have you been taking the medication consistently since last time?"

"Yes…well, for the most part," I told her. "I have been really good about taking them in the morning, but I still sometimes forget at night. After we met last time, I followed your advice of setting a reminder alarm for the evening. That really helped, but I have been slipping lately. Guess I need to go back to that practice."

About Face

Dr. Ted said, "Thanks for telling me the truth. That's what I'm looking for. Setting the reminder again is a good Baby Step. I really hope you will take a moment and reflect on how well you have done since we met. While you are not at your goal yet, you have taken a number of very impactful Baby Steps and your body is thanking you through the very significant improvements you are seeing.

"We know that taking the medication more consistently has helped, but frankly I believe that 85% of the changes are due to your choosing to do things a different way. Two of my favorite sayings are that, with type 2 diabetes, 'food is the strongest drug you put in your body' and 'exercise is the best medicine.'

"Combine this with better sleep and stress control and you are literally adding years to your life and life to your years. If we plotted your health through your life in the last three months, the line, which was going down steadily, has now turned and moved from worsening to improving. From an 'inside your body' perspective, your body is actually functioning like a younger and more vital body. You could say that you *decreased* in age from a health perspective since I saw you last time.

"Here's my bias about your numbers, Joe. While they are an important report card of your current state of health, they are not our primary focus. You will notice that, unlike a lot of doctors, I do not encourage you to set your vision on the numbers because they are actually lagging indicators of the choices you are making and the actions you are taking.

"It is the choices and the actions that are the key. They come first, the numbers follow. They let you know how well what you are trying is working. Focus on the Baby Steps and creating the life that inspires and motivates you. If you do this, the numbers will take care of themselves."

I thought what a refreshing way to look at the numbers.

She went on, "As you continue making progress, a possibility that I think will entice you – and it is just a possibility – is that you might very well get to the point where you can earn your way off of your medication."

I was excited about this news. "Really!? That's possible?"

"Yes. There is increasing evidence that, for some people, if we catch diabetes early, it can not only be controlled, but you may get to the place where your insulin supply and your body's uptake of blood sugar reach a healthy balance without taking pills. Remember, what is the strongest 'drug' you put in your body?"

"Food," I answered.

"Right, *food*. The best medicine?"

"Exercise.*"

"You've got it!" she responded with enthusiasm.

"So it makes sense that, as you make better choices, the need for pills will reduce. From the strides you have made so far, I think you may be a candidate for that – but let's not get ahead of ourselves."

I was delighted, "OK, Dr. Ted, but I am including that for my vision – that I am pill free."

"That's a good one, Joe. The other targets that will tell us you are nearing that point is when your fasting blood sugar is less than 100, your glucose after eating averages less than 140 and your hemoglobin A1c is less than 5.6."

I responded, "I can actually see that as a possibility now. *That* inspires me."

We explored more aspects of my choices and actions. She asked me what I thought were some of the challenges that were holding me back or stopping me from making progress. One that immediately came to mind was that I had a family history of diabetes that I could not do anything about and the fact that my circle of friends didn't share my new lifestyle. I told her, "My buddies still want to go out for pizza and beer every week or to watch football at the bar."

Dr. Ted said, "While you can't choose your genes and family history, I believe that 80% of developing type 2 diabetes is environmental. I have had patients who belong to families where three of the brothers and sisters get it and five do not. The difference? The choices and actions they make with food, exercise, sleep, and stress, to name some key ones.

"Being predisposed is not the same as being a Victim of your family's past. As for your friends, there are probably some choices you are going to have to face. You may need to consider how often you do things with them. You may decide to go against the flow and eat and drink differently from the group. While it may be difficult, as a Creator, remember that you are at choice as to what you are putting into your body, regardless of what family and friends are doing.

"You have one huge thing going for you, it sounds like, and that is how your wife has gotten on board. Perhaps your friends don't have to be all or nothing. Joining a walking club or a mountain climbing club will introduce you to some new friends with different priorities. That doesn't mean you don't spend some time with your old friends, but now you have a blend, and some new influence in your life."

I reflected over the first months after I was diagnosed. I had felt victimized by the way my friends and family acted towards me, and towards their own health. I felt much more empowered now. I didn't have to make the same choices they did in order to spend time with them. It might seem easier to go along with them, but ultimately it wasn't worth the consequences.

Dr. Ted leaned back and looked me in the eye. "I really want to complement you on your forward progress and momentum, Joe. I hope you will take time each day to appreciate how far you have come and to be grateful for your progress and the people in your life that are making the changes with you as you achieve new states of health and well-being. It is hard to be bitter, frustrated, and negative when you are appreciating the gifts that we are given in our lives.

"That said, I want to continue with our current course of treatment medically and to see you again in three months. I will have Marianne come in to sit down with you and, together, you and she can talk through the Baby Steps that you commit to between now and the next appointment.

"The idea of Baby Steps cannot be overstated here, Joe. Health will emerge over time and from taking lots and lots of Baby Steps. Keep up the good work!"

Marianne came back in soon after Dr. Ted left the room. She sat and looked over my chart. "Okay, let's set out some Baby Steps for you."

I interjected, "Didn't you say the last class topic would be Baby Steps? "

"Yes, it is," she answered. "Obviously I will go into more depth in the class, but let me ask you, do you remember the FISBE of a Creator Orientation?"

"Sure," I said, "It is so important to me that I have put your handout of both orientations next my mirror in the bathroom. That way I am reminded to start each day by focusing on what I want, rather than reacting to what I don't want."

"That's excellent, Joe. What is the behavioral part of the Creator Orientation?" she quizzed.

"Oh, yeah – the behavior in FISBE is Baby Steps."

Marianne responded, "That's how we make forward progress – it is all about taking those Baby Steps."

We then came up with several. First and foremost, I was to keep up with my making the choices and taking the actions on food, activity, sleep, and stress. I said, "I'm a little bored with walking."

Marianne asked, "What else could you do?"

After some brainstorming, I decided to look into a hiking club in the area that could help me prepare for the family reunion. I also committed to buying my wife and myself a used bicycle and begin riding, which is something I loved to do when I was younger. Maybe we could even get bikes for the kids and do some weekend rides as a family.

"Any other Baby Steps you want to set for yourself?" Marianne asked.

"Yes, there's one more. The current bowling league season is coming to an end and I think I'll take a break and not sign up for the next one. A lot of the enjoyment was eating pizza or burgers and drinking beer together. I am sure they will be disappointed, but honestly, I know that several of them are in trouble with their health, so maybe they will consider what they are doing to themselves also. I can see my friends at church and maybe I will invite them to walk or ride with me. I am sure doing this will help me make better choices about my eating and drinking."

Marianne patted me on the back as I stood up, "Deciding who you spend time with, and what you do together, can be very challenging. I'm so glad to hear that you're operating from a perspective of empowerment."

The Last Class, a New Era

While there was a sense of excitement among the class members to share success stories and receive supportive coaching regarding setbacks as well, there was a subtle sadness floating over the group.

Marianne stood up at the front of the room and said, "I have so enjoyed working with you for the past five sessions. As you know, tonight is our last night together. However, I do want to invite you to our ongoing alumni group. You are welcome to attend any time you choose. I attend myself, as another Creator with diabetes. As a single woman, the support I give and receive is a critical part of my own health and well-being. I would love to keep up with your progress through your participation in the group."

Ram spoke up, "At the risk of making you sound like a Rescuer, I want to say that your instruction has changed my life." A number of people spoke up in affirmation.

Marianne smiled, "I'll take that in the spirit it was intended. Seeing the difference in how many of you approach your diabetes - and life in general - in more empowered and resourceful ways is the payoff for me. I love this work. Creating, challenging, and coaching is a great way to live.

"In this last class, I'd like to do something a little different. I'd like you to pick a partner so that we can do an exercise." People paired off around the room. I turned toward Ram and said, "Want to work together?"

He did, so we shifted our chairs toward each other. Marianne continued her instruction. She had the Dynamic Tension diagram on the board. Underneath "Current Reality" she wrote the word *Supports* on one side and *Inhibits* on the other.

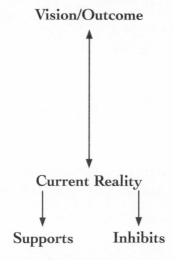

Vision/Outcome

Current Reality

Supports   **Inhibits**

"Working together, I'd like you to make a list of what supports you, or what is helpful, in creating your envisioned outcome of health and well-being. It is helpful to look at facts, feelings, observable behavior, and self-talk.

"Similarly, I want you to list problems or obstacles that need to be dealt with in order to go after your outcome. These are what we call the inhibitors. Assessing both your supports, as well as inhibitors, is a vital practice. Someone once said, 'what determines our destiny is not the hand we are dealt, but how to play the hand – and the way to play the hand is to see reality for what it is and to act accordingly.' Seeing the full range of supporting and inhibiting factors in your current reality is crucial."

Ram and I got to work. By the time Marianne called us back as a group, I had written quite a list. Under "Supports" I had:

* Attending this class
* Exercising regularly
* Eating fewer refined and simple carbs/sugars
* Checking blood sugar at least 2 times/day
* Setting specific goals that are exciting to me and require fitness
* Lois is supportive
* JJ and Lisa are more accepting and understanding than ever

Under "Inhibits" I had:

* Doubts about sticking with it after the class ends
* Kids still eating junk food, which tempts me
* My closest circle of friends is not very supportive
* Fear of failure or setbacks

Marianne asked if anyone wanted to share some of what was on their own lists. A number of people read from their lists, many with similar themes to mine.

After those who wanted to share were finished, Marianne said, "Again, avoiding denial and telling the truth about current reality is critical. Only then can you plan effective Baby Steps that will take you toward your desired outcome.

"Part of the power in committing to and taking Baby Steps is that we build our pathway, which emerges over time, through small, incremental actions. We can easily get overwhelmed when we set big, hairy, audacious outcomes and goals – like creating health and well-being – if we try and figure everything out before we start taking action."

Many in the class nodded. I said to Ram, "Yeah, I always get overwhelmed by the hairy ones!"

Marianne said, "There are three criteria for effective Baby Steps." She wrote *1) short term* on the board. "Baby Steps," she explained, "are always short term. Can someone give me an example of a goal that is not a Baby Step?"

A woman in the back said, "I'm going to exercise everyday for the rest of my life." The class laughed.

Marianne said, "Can you feel how the statement 'the rest of my life' feels like a huge burden? When you put an unrealistic timeframe on a step, it's not a Baby Step.

"The second criterion is that the baby step is also something that you can do." She wrote, *2) doable* on the board. She said, "Baby Steps are actionable, meaning they are things you can actually do. The last criterion is equally important." She wrote, *3) they are 100% yours to do.* You can only commit to your own baby steps. You cannot commit for another person.

"To say, 'I am going to eat a breakfast with less than 30 grams of carbohydrates that I like for the next 14 days,' meets all three criteria. To say, 'My family will start each day with a healthy breakfast,' does not meet the criteria, because you cannot control your family's choices."

That hit home for me. I realized that I kept trying to change the eating habits of my wife and children. And, of course, I can't.

Marianne continued, "Every time you take a Baby Step, one of three things is going to happen." First, and most often, it is going to be just that – a Baby Step that produces incremental forward progress. We would call that a victory.

"The second is that you take a Baby Step and it ends up being a step back. This could be a mistake or making a choice that does not serve your envisioned outcome, so it moves you away from your goal. When this happens, you learn from it and then make the next choice. It's a slip up, not a give up.

"The third possibility is an exciting one. You never know when a Baby Step is going to turn into a giant leap of forward progress or a breakthrough that would not have happened had you not taken the Baby Step.

"For example, in my own journey, a couple years after my diagnosis, I set the intention of learning what it would take to become a diabetes educator. I did lots of research. This led me to realize that I could accomplish this outcome, so I set the Baby Step of applying to the program within 14 days, which I did, and got accepted. I was working full-time, but kept taking classes which ultimately led to my graduation – one Baby Step at a time. On the journey, one of the seemingly hundreds of Baby Steps in my study and training was to seek out an internship with a doctor.

"One particular Baby Step was to approach Dr. Ted about an internship. She was new to the area and had just opened her practice. While it felt like a Baby Step at the time, going to meet her about an internship turned out to be a giant leap forward for me. Actually, I didn't know to call it a Baby Step then, since I learned this approach and language from her. The truth is, I would not be here today with you had I not taken that step."

Ram said to me, "Meeting Marianne was that kind of Baby Step that turned out to be a giant leap for me."

I agreed. It was certainly the case for me as well.

A Surprise Ending

Marianne then said she had a surprise for us. "We like to close the class series by hearing from one of the graduates who has really put what you have learned here into practice. So, I would like to ask our friend Mark to share a bit of his story."

As he stood and walked toward the front of the room, I immediately recognized him as the man

I met in the class session on adopting a Creator Orientation. He smiled broadly and slowly looked around the room. "I am so honored to be here tonight and share my story with you.

"I was first diagnosed with diabetes over ten years ago. Even though I am insulin-dependent with my type 2 diabetes, I am grateful to say that my life is rich and full and healthier than I ever imagined.

"Back then, even though I had many of the classic symptoms, I didn't recognize I had a problem at first. When I had trouble seeing, my eye doctor made it abundantly clear that I had to get to the doctor. I was really scared at the time. There wasn't the breadth of information available back then, either.

"Unfortunately, my doctor at the time wasn't much help - and I was not exactly an empowered patient. He gave me the usual, 'Lose weight and exercise' speech, but I didn't really understand how diet and exercise directly impacted my disease. I didn't know that within thirty minutes of eating carbohydrates, for example, more sugar was put into my blood stream. And exercise? It seemed like a horrible imposition to work that into my schedule. I had no idea that through movement I was burning up excess sugar in my system.

"In the beginning, I worked really hard at managing my diabetes. I would do what I was supposed to. You know, check my numbers, eat well, and exercise. I would get a good report from my doctor and then let up because it all seemed to be going well. This went on for a couple of years. I got sick and tired of being on that roller coaster.

"It wasn't until I found my way to Dr. Ted that I began to see all of the connections between my ways of thinking, my behavior, and my health. I will never forget the second time I went to see her and met Marianne for the first time. She told me she was starting this class and invited me to attend."

Mark smiled at Marianne, "I'm proud to have been in that first class. And I didn't get her information a moment too soon. I shudder to think what my health, my entire life, would be without my re-framing how I relate to diabetes.

"I got to meet some of you when I sat in on the class in which you were introduced to the idea of a Creator Orientation. The shift began happening in my life the night I really, really got that I could create and live a life of meaning, purpose, and passion – and a life of health – by focusing on what I want, rather than seeing my diabetes as a problem to solve and react to.

"While I still have my days of wishing I didn't have to take insulin, most of the time I am focused on positive things, like all the wonderful food I get to eat and learning new ways of preparing nutritious dishes. I went from walking to jogging to running. Two weeks ago I completed my first half-marathon. I focus on the joy of being with my children, my grandchildren, and friends. I can't tell you how happy I am that my family has not only been supportive, but my kids are raising their kids with health in mind. I am convinced we are on our way to breaking the cycle of passing diabetes on from generation to generation."

Mark paused and took a drink of water.

"This class and Dr. Ted have taught and prepared me to relate to my diabetes through TED*. There is much, much less drama these days. I am a Creator with diabetes who is supported by my family, the new friends I have made who share this way of living with me, and a wonderful medical team that serve me as Coaches and Challengers.

"One of the most liberating parts of this teaching, for me, has been the concept of Baby Steps. I make one choice at a time. Checking my blood sugar is a Baby Step. Deciding what to eat is a Baby Step. Getting out in nature for a hike or playing in the park with my grandkids is a choice and a Baby Step. You don't have to have a huge complicated plan to make this all work. It's about creating a life of health and wellbeing one Baby Step at a time. I no longer feel so frustrated by unrealistic expectations. I'm not knocked off my feet with guilt when I'm not perfect. I know it's actually possible to succeed."

Mark got a sheepish grin on his face. "I can be a little obsessive at times, but I want to share with you something that has helped give me a sense of accomplishment." He reached down and picked up a regular sized piece of paper, then unfolded it to reveal a long spread sheet he had made for himself.

He said proudly, "This is my Baby Step Chart where I track my numbers, my caloric intake, my exercise sessions, and other small steps I take toward meeting my current goals."

Ram leaned over and whispered, "I made one of those for myself too, but I was too embarrassed to admit it!"

We both chuckled, while I raised my hand, "Mark, I say use whatever method works for you!"

The group nodded in agreement. Marianne jumped in, "Thank you Mark for showing us your chart. I encourage you all to create ways that affirm your progress."

A woman near the front said, "It reminds me of the sticker chart I used with my son when he was growing up. I think I need to make a sticker chart for myself."

Mark said, "Now, I know that Marianne tells us not to obsess on numbers, but I do want to brag a little! When I was first diagnosed, I weighed 20% more than I do today, and my A1c was almost 10. Now I have an average A1c that is typically around 6.5. Yes, I have my diabetes, but it does not have me. "

We spontaneously clapped at his declaration. Mark took a mock bow and beamed.

His statement reverberated in my mind: I have diabetes, but it doesn't have me.

Mark continued, "I want to close by saying that I feel better today than I did in the years before my diagnosis. Back then I confused not feeling sick with being healthy. I'm sure you've heard others say that diabetes can be seen as a gift in the form of a wake-up call that can extend the quality and length of our lives. Well, that is certainly the truth of my experience. Living life as a Creator with diabetes has enriched my life beyond measure. I want to take this opportunity to thank Marianne for the amazing impact she's had on my life, and to thank you for letting me share."

Mark then paused and gestured toward the back of the room. "And to you, Dr. Ted," he said with a broad smile to the doctor who had silently slipped in during his sharing. "I am so grateful."

We once again erupted in applause and several shouted, "Hurray for Marianne!" "Let's hear it for Dr. Ted!"

As Mark took his seat, Dr. Ted walked gracefully to the front and stood next to Marianne.

Dr. Ted smiled, "Thank you, Mark, for sharing your story. You – and all of you," she said to the room, "are what it's all about. As Mark is a testimony to, we create outcomes by engaging in the 3-step dance of Dynamic Tension, which is the ongoing steps of three questions: 'What do I want?' 'What do I have?' and 'What's next?'

"It is a dance we do every day. Setting daily Baby Steps is one of the primary disciplines of creating an inspiring and motivating life while managing your diabetes. By staying focused on adopting a Creator Orientation and the TED* role of being a Creator; engaging with the disease as a Challenger that is sparking learning and, in the long run, health; and developing a support system around you and using one another and your healthcare professionals as Coaches, I have absolute confidence in your evolving capability to live a fulfilling life, and in the process you will become a very positive influence on those around you."

Marianne thanked Dr. Ted, turned to the group and, with a little quiver in her voice, said, "Let me just say that I've thoroughly enjoyed working with you all. I hope to see you at the alumni group, if that is what will help you create your envisioned outcome. Being in a supportive community like this can do wonders."

As I looked around the class for the last time, I smiled and said goodbye to a number of people. Ram and I walked out of the community center together. I realized in the process of the last few months, that we had actually become friends. We were partners on the path toward creating optimum health.

Ram lightly patted my shoulder and said, "See ya, buddy. I am definitely planning on going to the support group starting next week. I hope to see you there."

"You can count on it."

EPILOGUE

Attending the Family Reunion

It's the first night of the reunion, and nothing has turned out as I had feared. In the last nine months, my anxiety about attending our family reunion slowly turned into excited anticipation.

So much has changed—for the better—since my initial diagnosis of diabetes. It certainly wasn't an easy time. Don't get me wrong. It was quite a challenge to stay on track with my Baby Steps and to address all of the changes I ultimately needed to make to meet my diabetes goals. My diagnosis turned out to be a wake-up call for me to embrace life on a completely different level.

Lois, the kids, and I had headed off to the reunion with me twenty-five pounds lighter, and Lois twelve pounds lighter than when we received the invitation. My numbers have decreased so significantly (my HgbA1c is 6.0) that Dr. Ted told me I was in the "prediabetic" range. I'm still taking medication, but Dr. Ted says at this point it is really my choice whether I go off or not, but it is not hurting anything and is safe if I stay on. Rather than obsessing on these issues, I'm much more focused on the exciting process of creating health in my life.

We ended up driving, due in part to my reluctance to initially commit to attending the reunion. But also because we've been doing so much better as a family, we all decided that a drive across the country would be a great family experience. And it has turned out that way. We took an extra week to visit historical sites, climb a few hills at national parks, and see some friends we have in states along the way. My son and I now share a great love for digital photography and hill climbing, and we got some great shots from the peaks that we climbed along the way.

Now that we're at the reunion, it's turning out to be more fun than I ever imagined. My cousin set up the reunion at a rural combination motel and campground that caters to people and groups that come for reunions or to fish or to hike in the nearby mountains. It's a really comfortable location that feels very homey.

It has been great to get reconnected with four generations of family members. My grandmother is in her nineties, but still alert and able to make us all laugh with her tales of the "good ol' days." My mother passed away when I was in college, but my dad and my step-mother are here. I have vowed to get together with them more often, even though they live quite a distance from us now. My sister and our cousins are here—with a slew of teen-agers in tow. None of the young adults have married or have children yet, but it probably won't be long before we welcome the next generation into our fold.

We met tonight at a large shelter that is nothing more than a big slab of concrete with a half dozen picnic tables, and heavy duty grills at each end and plenty of room for folding chairs. As soon as my cousin Frank, the "exercise freak" cousin saw me, he slapped me on the back and said, "Joe, there is less of you here than I have seen in a long time. You look pretty healthy, dude!"

I smiled, but inside I thought that hearing that comment from Frank made the whole trip worth-while. I told him about my journey of the past year and the gift that my diabetes turned out to be. I was so into my story that I didn't notice until the end that Frank was grinning ear-to-ear.

Frank said, "Do you know why I have been so focused on my own health for the last decade? Because ten years ago I was diagnosed with predia-betes and I began making choices that would steer my life in a different direction. As I did, I discov-ered that I really love being outdoors and paying attention to what I put into my body. That diag-nosis was my wake-up call as well."

Since Frank and I hadn't talked much over the years, it didn't surprise me that he hadn't had a chance to share his diagnosis with me. (After all, how many of us want to announce to relatives we see occasionally, "Oh, by the way, I've been diagnosed with diabetes!") Had he shared it with me, maybe it could have served as an indicator to me to take better care of my health. I wasn't open to that kind of conversation back then. All of a sudden, Frank seemed like a fellow-companion, rather than someone I kept at arm's length.

After dinner, the entire family gathered around in a large circle around the shelter to share stories and get up to date on what was going on in everyone's lives. Frank and I described our situations and we discussed how diabetes has been a part of our family system. Some of the other cousins expressed their surprise to learn how prevalent it has been. We all agreed to gather together in the morning before breakfast and the hike to check our fasting blood sugar levels. What I feared would be an embarrassing confession turned out to be the catalyst for an eye-opening conversation that may well help my relatives avoid developing full-blown diabetes.

That feels really good.

Right now, though, I need to get some good rest so I can wake up early. Having everyone see their numbers in the morning is going to be very interesting – and I am really looking forward to that hike. I bet the views from up there are amazing!

AFTERWORD

Little did I know that this would be the first book in applying *The Power of TED* (*The Empowerment Dynamic)* to various aspects of life. Indeed, little did I know that a few months after completing the writing of TED* in late 2005, I would receive the diagnosis of type 2 diabetes.

While Joe is a fictional character, some of his experience is based upon my own. When my doctor – upon whom Joe's first doctor is *not* based – first informed me of needing to confront diabetes, I initially rejected his suggestion of going on medication. I was convinced I could fight the disease through diet and exercise. I did, to a point (more on that in a moment).

In early 2007 I was invited to deliver one of the first TED* presentations and workshops to a leadership program in which one of the participants was Dr. Scott Conard. Participants in this graduate leadership program had been given *The Power of TED** in advance. I distinctly remember Scott telling me the positive impact the book had had in his life and medical practice.

Some months later, while sitting at my desk on Bainbridge Island, Washington, I received a call from Scott informing me that he was in Seattle attending a conference and wanted to know if we could have lunch – that day. Fatefully, I was free.

He took the ferry over and, during our lunch, I shared with him my diagnosis. I quickly learned that this was an area of specialty for him as a General Practitioner. As is his style, he proceeded to energetically diagram for me on the back of a napkin what was going on in my body when I ingested what he informed me was the most powerful drug that every person consumes – food.

Upon one of my visits to Dallas, Scott invited me to visit him at his office. It was during that visit that he first suggested we consider co-writing a book applying the ways of thinking, interacting, and taking action in TED* to this disease that affects millions upon millions of people around the world.

I wish I could say that I immediately agreed. I also wish I could say that I was taking an approach to my relationship with diabetes that reflected adopting a Creator Orientation. I didn't and I wasn't.

After a year or so of trying to manage on my own with marginal success, I capitulated with my doctor and agreed to take oral medication. With the addition of the medication, modest and inconsistent adjustments to what I ate, and a fairly conscientious increase of exercise, over the ensuing years I was able to keep my "numbers in range" in managing my diabetes.

I was fortunate in many regards. The diabetes was diagnosed early, thanks to having a healthcare plan that covered annual physical exams. My family physician and his team were supportive and informative when I had my regular checkups and blood work labs reviewed (though I can't say I always took advantage of what they offered). I had an extremely supportive spouse and family system. I have learned that many of these factors are not always the case for those who received the challenging news of having diabetes.

Even with all of those positive aspects of my experience, I just plodded along. I rode the roller coaster of results in the Victim Orientation. Diabetes was my Persecutor and I its Victim. For a time I would take focused action, the numbers would come down and – especially using the fact that I was taking medication as a Rescuer from the disease – I would slack off after seeing success. Of course, in slacking, the numbers would again increase. The good news is that they were still almost always "in range" for managing diabetes.

Then in early 2011, Donna (my wife and business partner) and I had an auspicious lunch conversation with Dr. Scott. About halfway through, he turned to me and asked, yet again, "When are we going to write that book on TED* and diabetes?" He then turned to Donna and said to her, "I have only been after him for years about this!"

To my own surprise I replied, "I'm ready. Let's do it."

After a month or so of framing our collaboration and outlining the initial storyline, the writing began. Then all kinds of serendipitous and synchronistic things started to happen. Roy M Carlisle, our remarkable editor and publishing consultant, who I knew was an insulin dependent type 2 diabetic, was a bit stunned when I ran the idea of the book by him (he thought we were going to write first on TED* in the workplace). But he immediately caught the vision. When I expressed interest in someone who could assist in the writing, he put me in touch with Carmen Renee Berry, who I was able to meet personally within a month when I "happened" to be in her area while working as an executive coach.

The "twin sisters" of serendipity and synchronicity continued – and still continue – to show up.

But something else happened. As we began to write, I realized that I was out of integrity with my own work. The realization gnawed at me as I came to see how much the managing and relating to my diabetes was rooted in that Victim Orientation.

I declared to Donna that I needed to – that I *chose to* – shift my focus to a Creator Orientation and that what I wanted was to create health in my life.

Within a couple of weeks, through a conversation that she had with a mutual friend, we learned about Take Shape for Life, a lifestyle program based on Dr. Wayne Andersen's book, *Habits of Health*[1].

It was another Baby Step of serendipity, as we found that the process utilized Robert Fritz's Creative Tension model as an organizing and mental framework.

The timing was perfect. We enrolled in the program and I began working with Kathryn Leslie, one of the Take Shape for Life health coaches. I engaged the Dynamic Tension between what I wanted and my current reality.

Optimal health became my focus. The envisioned outcome was defined by how I would know it when I created it, which was increased energy, vitality, well-being, and (as mundane as it might sound) fitting into the same size blue jeans as I wore in college.

Getting to a preferred weight was the first order of business. One of the major dietary changes was to eat (i.e. "fuel") with low glycemic food every 3 hours in order to even out the sugar/insulin process. Exercise took on a different rhythm and focus.

---

1   While having gained immensely from Dr. A's *Habits of Health*, the Take Shape for Life process and the support my health coach, this is not intended as an explicit endorsement of this specific program over others. There are numerous programs and processes that help individuals develop healthy lifestyles. My encouragement is to find one that speaks to you.

The results of the shift to a Creator Orientation in which my focus is on creating optimal health have surprised even me. While this focus and the Baby Steps that I take will be a lifelong process – and the envisioned outcome is not yet fully realized – I was pleasantly surprised when, after six months of taking action, I received the blood work lab report that indicated that my A1C was "normal for a non-diabetic."

When I texted the results to Dr. Scott, he immediately replied "You are now undiabetic!"

Whether that continues to be the case for me remains to be seen. I know that the changes in lifestyle that I have committed to will be lifelong and that I will need to work daily in taking Baby Steps, making conscious and healthy choices, and living with gratitude for the "wake up call" to health empowerment of my diagnosis.

Whatever your situation, adopting a Creator Orientation can make a difference in your life and in the lives of those around you – whether you are the one with diabetes or it is a loved one with the disease.

It is our intention that this little story provide hope and encouragement for anyone who is dealing with the Challenger of diabetes. One of the things we know about diabetes is that, with conscious and concerted effort, this disease can be avoided, delayed and/or slowed in its progression. In some cases, such as mine, it may even be able to be reversed.

While the advent of a disease such as diabetes may not avoidable, due to genetics or other factors, the choice for health empowerment is just that – a choice. What determines our response is not the hand we are dealt, but how we play the hand.

This book is not intended to be a "primer" on diabetes. There is plenty of good information available from a wide variety of resources on the medical science and physiology of diabetes.

In fact, I am not an expert in the science – not by a long shot. Dr. Scott and Roy (who is one of the most knowledgeable and "activated patients" you would ever want to know) are much more knowledgeable than me.

This I *do* know: by focusing on creating health, making healthy choices and taking daily Baby Steps, vitality and wellbeing are attainable. We may not be able to cure what ails us, but we can heal in remarkable ways.

> **To the Creator in you!**
> **David Emerald**
> **Bainbridge Island, Washington**

APPENDIX A

Seven Daily Practices:

* **Intention Setting and Baby Steps** – Setting intentions on a daily basis is incredibly empowering and important. Begin each day by choosing 1-3 Baby Step actions that will support you in creating health in your life. It might be walking an extra 10 minutes or trying a new recipe or coming back for one more class and/or the support group. Remember, Baby Steps are things you can do that day that are also actionable and yours to do.

* **Three Hour "Time out!"** – Use your watch, computer, telephone or any kind of alarm to go off every 3 hours. When the alarm sounds, there are two things to do: first, reflect on which Orientation you have been operating from during that time period. Is there a need to make a shift happen? Second, have something that is

low glycemic to eat – a few almonds, an apple, a slice of whole grain bread. There is increasing evidence that, by "fueling" yourself every 3 hours, you help even out your blood sugar and insulin.

* **See Yourself (and Everyone) as a Creator** – Re-member that you have the capacity to create outcomes, like optimal health, in your life and to choose your responses to life circumstances. It is all about choice and you are responsibly (response-able) for the choices you make. You are a Creator who is managing your diabetes through your choices, you are not a diabetic.

* **Ask: What am I Learning?** – This will help you keep your life experiences—including your diabetes—in perspective as a Challenger that sparks learning and growth, rather than as a Persecutor to react to. Welcome conscious, constructive Challengers into your life who help you learn and stretch in attaining your envisioned outcomes.

* **Leverage Your Support System** – There is no weakness in seeking support as a Creator, because you know that the power and responsibility for creating and choosing is ultimately your own. When you are stuck or unclear about something, ask for the support of a Coach, whether the person taking on that role is a healthcare or personal development professional, a trusted friend, or someone who shares similar challenges and questions as you do. Finding a diabetes

support group can also be an excellent resource.

* **Speak to What you Want** – By focusing on what you want (rather than what you don't want) will keep you more consistently rooted in a Creator Orientation.

* **End-of-Day Reflection** – Take a few minutes at the end of the day to reflect on how the day went. Did you move closer to—or further away from—your intended outcome? Did you make healthy choices? If not, what can you do the following day to make new choices that support you?

By applying these seven daily practices, you will be increasing awareness, developing new patterns and habits of behavior, and creating optimal health – Baby Step by Baby Step!

APPENDIX B

The Seven Healers

Do you want to live a healthy, fulfilling life? This is not just a measure of our physical condition; beliefs, values, and habits that shape every area of our lives. The Seven Healers are seven specific ingredients that we need in order to survive and thrive in this life, and they are essential to managing, delaying or even reversing diabetes.

1. **Air** – You can only live minutes without air. Your body takes in oxygen, and eliminates waste and toxins through breathing. While quick, shallow breaths are toxic and are associated with stress in our body, slow deep breaths increase concentration, lower stress hormone levels, and facilitate a feeling of calmness and peace. Two of the best things you can do to regain the full function of your lungs is to *become aware of your breathing* and *begin practicing deep-breathing exercises*.

2. **Water** – Every cell in our body is a small lake of water. In addition to sustaining your cells, water is a major detoxifying and cleansing agent in your body. Without adequate amounts of fresh water daily symptoms such as muscle aches, joint pain, headaches, fatigue, and soreness can begin to appear. Don't wait until you are thirsty to drink. Keep yourself hydrated, and you'll keep yourself out of trouble.

3. **Sleep** – Sleep is vital to every aspect of your life. You need seven and a half to nine hours of sleep a night for optimal health. That's about fifty-four hours per week and includes powernaps and extended siestas on the weekend. When you sleep, you cycle through specific stages throughout the night: non-REM (NR) 1 - 3, and REM sleep. Each stage allows your body and mind to repair and heal itself. With adequate sleep, you can achieve hormonal balance, strengthen your mind and immune system, and reduce fatigue and irritability.

4. **Food** – Food is the strongest drug you put in your body. While making unhealthy food choices will diminish the quality and quantity of your life, healthy choices will enhance it. Since the body breaks down food into three major forms—carbohydrates, fats, and proteins—it's important to get all these nutrients at each meal along with vital micronutrients and adequate fiber.

5. **Play** — Play is the best medicine for your body, and it doesn't have to be strenuous or boring to be beneficial. Every activity counts and adds value to your life. Regular activity reduces toxicity by activating the lymphatic system. It also reduces the symptoms of anxiety and depression, balances stress hormones, strengthens your circulatory system, and activates your receptors on cells that effectively help lower your blood sugar and triglyceride levels. Aim to play at least every other day for twenty to thirty minutes; you will reap the rich rewards that follow!

6. **Relationships** — Healthy, loving relationships are vital for a meaningful life. Clearly, the company we keep powerfully impacts our direction and destiny. Select friends living the life you imagine. Remember better relationships start with your relationship with yourself. Finding forgiveness, acceptance, and love sets you free to be all you can be and build relationships that are life-giving!

7. **Purpose** — Having purpose, a reason for living—it is the "why" behind what we do. Without it, we have no direction, no meaning, and no fulfillment. You have a unique destiny. Discovering your purpose begins with and finds full expression in letting go of being a "knower" and embracing a new way of living as a "learner" living not in the 1 percent that you know but in the 99% percent that you don't know. It is in this

that you will find the joy and fulfillment that you seek. As you trust with all your heart and lean not on your own understanding, your path of purpose will emerge and become clear.

＊ Excerpted from *The Seven Healers*, by Scott Conard M.D. For more information visit www.rapha7ven.com.

GLOSSARY

I. Diabetes Terms

A1C – a test used to track how well a person is taking care of their diabetes, as well as diagnose diabetes. An A1C test measures how much glucose (sugar, converted from carbohydrates in food) has been sticking to your red blood cells over the past 3 months. The American Diabetes Association standards advise that an A1C of 6.5% or higher is considered diabetes; an A1C of 5.7%--6.4% is considered prediabetes. The higher your A1C, the more you will experience health complications from diabetes. A1C is also called hemoglobin A1C or glycosylated (gly-KOH-sih-lay-ted) hemoglobin. Hemoglobin (HEE-mo-glo-bin) is the part of a red blood cell that carries oxygen to the cells.

A1C to Glucose (mg/dl) Table

People with diabetes may test daily with a blood glucose meter and also test quarterly for an A1C result. Since the two tests provide results in different measurements, this handy chart shows you the A1C equivalent for average daily blood glucose results. Knowing how the two types of tests relate can be helpful in managing diabetes.

The higher your A1C and blood glucose levels, the more likely you are to experience health complications from diabetes.

A1C	eAG	
%	mg/dl	mmol/l
6	126	7.0
6.5	140	7.8
7	154	8.6
7.5	169	9.4
8	183	10.1
8.5	197	10.9
9	212	11.8
9.5	226	12.6
10	240	13.4

blood glucose – also called blood sugar, glucose is a form of sugar (converted from the carbohydrates in food) and your body's main source of energy. Diabetes disrupts the body's ability to process food into energy, and when blood glucose fluctuates too high or too low (and stays out of normal range) your body experiences health complications.

blood glucose level – the amount of glucose (sugar, converted from the carbohydrates in food) in a blood sample. People with diabetes have blood glucose levels that frequently rise and fall (like a roller coaster), and the swings can cause mild to severe health complications.

Blood glucose is measured in milligrams per deciliter, mg/dl, or millimoles per litre (mmol/l).

blood glucose meter – a small, portable medical device used to check blood glucose levels. Using a blood glucose meter to test before/after meals and exercise tells you how your activities impact your blood glucose levels so you can make choices, and changes, throughout each day.

borderline diabetes – prediabetes or impaired glucose tolerance; you may not have been officially diagnosed, but your body is showing signs of developing diabetes. This is also called prediabetes or metabolic syndrome. It represents the period between normal functioning and formally qualifying for the diagnosis of diabetes.

The American Diabetes Association considers an A1C test result of 5.7%–6.4% prediabetes.

diabetes mellitus (MELL-ih-tus) – means your body no longer successfully processes food into energy—like it is supposed to—and has to get help through lifestyle changes and medication. The balance between what is taken in and what is needed is out of balance and the ability of the pancreas to force the process has been compromised by lack of receptiveness or lack of the ability to produce enough insulin. A persistent illness, diabetes has serious health consequences when not managed or treated. Diabetes is a growing worldwide health epidemic.

Different stages of diabetes include:

Prediabetes: A condition in which blood glucose levels are higher than normal, but not high enough for a diagnosis of diabetes. This is the period during which the body has the possibility of recovering and not moving ahead to full blown diabetes if changes are made in the energy balance. Making healthy diet and activity choices can delay or prevent diabetes, and reduce health complications.

Type 1 diabetes: The pancreas doesn't make insulin, which is a hormone necessary to convert food into energy. If you have type 1 diabetes, you must take insulin every day (via injection or pump).

Type 2 diabetes: Either the pancreas does not make enough insulin or the body is unable to respond to insulin correctly. People with type 2 diabetes manage their illness with medication (pills), or insulin, along with changing diet and activity choices.

Gestational diabetes: Some women develop blood sugars that are in the range of people with diabetes during pregnancy that resolve or go back to normal after the baby is delivered. These women are at increased risk of developing diabetes later in their life. Making healthy diet and activity choices can delay or prevent diabetes, and reduce health complications.

fasting blood glucose test – a blood test for glucose that is done after 8 hours or more of not eating (fasting). Why no food before the test? If your blood glucose is outside the normal range when you haven't eaten, it's a sign your body needs help to convert food to energy.

glycemic index (GI) (gly-SEE-mik) – a number assigned to carbohydrate containing food to provide an idea of how quickly and how dramatically the food will raise the blood glucose level. Being aware of which foods raise or lower blood glucose may help you make balanced food choices and manage your diabetes.

hypoglycemia (hy-po-gly-SEE-mee-uh) – hypo meaning low, glycemia meaning blood glucose. This number varies for different people at different times in their lives. For people who have no prediabetes or diabetes, hypoglycemia symptoms may occur when the blood glucose is less than 70 mg/dl (4mmol/l). People with prediabetes they may not develop symptoms until the blood sugar is even lower, sometimes as low as 40 or 50. In people with chronic diabetes, symptoms often develop with a rapid lowering of the blood sugar, even though the number may be as high as 110. Hypoglycemia becomes dangerous when the individual goes low enough that vital organs such as the brain, which depends almost entirely on glucose as fuel, do not have enough fuel to operate normally. Hypoglycemia can be especially challenging for people with type 1 diabetes or anyone using insulin, because if left untreated, low blood glucose can lead to unconsciousness.

Signs of low blood glucose include hunger, nervousness, shakiness, perspiration, dizziness or light-headedness, sleepiness, and confusion. Hypoglycemia is treated by consuming carbohydrate-rich foods or drinks such as a glucose tablet or juice. You may also treat hypoglycemia with an injection of glucagon, if the person is unconscious or unable to swallow.

impaired fasting glucose (IFG) – also called pre-diabetes, your body is showing signs that it is not processing insulin properly (impaired fasting glucose), and you are at increased risk for developing type 2 diabetes. Impaired Fasting Glucose levels may range from 100 mg/dl (5.5 mmol/l) to 125 mg/dl (6.9 mmol/l), and are a sign to make lifestyle changes to prevent or delay the onset of diabetes and associated health complications.

insulin – a hormone that helps the body use glucose for energy. Cells in the pancreas make insulin (necessary to convert food to energy). When the body cannot make enough insulin, you may need to take insulin by injection or via an insulin pump.

insulin resistance – the body's inability to respond to and use insulin properly. Insulin is a hormone (from the pancreas) needed to convert the food you eat into energy. You may be more likely to develop insulin resistance if you are overweight, have high blood pressure, and have high levels of fat in your blood.

metabolic syndrome – a group of risk factors that—alone and in combination—increase your chance for health problems, including heart disease, diabetes and strokes. Conditions likely to increase your risk for health complications include being overweight, high triglycerides, low HDL (good) cholesterol, high blood pressure and high fasting blood glucose (prediabetes). Habits that also impact metabolic syndrome include smoking, and little or no exercise. You can delay or prevent metabolic (or prediabetes) risk factors from becoming serious health issues with help from your health care team and a lifelong commitment to healthy living.

metformin (met-FOR-min) – an oral medicine commonly used to treat type 2 diabetes. Metformin lowers blood glucose by reducing the amount of glucose produced by the liver and helping the body respond better to the insulin made in the pancreas. Belongs to the class of medicines called biguanides.

(Brand names: Glucophage, Glucophage XR; an ingredient in Glucovance)

mg/dl - milligrams (MILL-ih-grams) per deciliter (DESS-ih-lee-tur). In the United States, blood glucose test results are reported as mg/dl. Medical journals and other countries use millimoles per liter (mmol/l). To convert to mg/dl from mmol/l, multiply by 18. Example: 10 mmol/l x 18 = 180 mg/dl.

pancreas (PAN-kree-us) – a gland integral to digestion. The pancreas makes insulin (a hormone necessary to convert food into energy). The pancreas is located behind the lower part of the stomach and is about the size of a hand. Damage to the pancreas (from inflammation or a genetic disorder like cystic fibrosis) can cause diabetes or increase diabetes symptoms.

peripheral neuropathy (puh-RIF-uh-rul ne-ROP-uh-thee) – nerve damage that affects the feet, legs, or hands. Peripheral neuropathy causes pain, numbness, or a tingling feeling, and is a complication in poorly controlled diabetes.

prediabetes – a condition in which blood glucose levels are higher than normal but are not high enough for a diagnosis of diabetes. Prediabetes is also called impaired glucose tolerance, impaired fasting glucose and borderline diabetes.

The American Diabetes Association estimates that there are 79 million people in the United States who have prediabetes. Studies suggest that even during prediabetes, the body can suffer health complications. People with prediabetes are at increased risk for developing type 2 diabetes and for heart disease and stroke. An A1C of 5.7%--6.4% is considered prediabetes, as in a fasting glucose level between 100 and 125.

self-management – in diabetes, self-management is the daily approach to managing diabetes. Self-management includes meal planning, physical activity, blood glucose monitoring, taking diabetes medicines, handling episodes of illness and of low and high blood glucose, managing diabetes when traveling, and more.

team management – an approach to treating diabetes. Medical care is provided by a team of health care professionals that specialize in medical concerns related to diabetes and its complications, including: a doctor, a dietitian, a diabetes educator, a personal trainer, eye and foot doctors, dermatologist, a neurologist (nerve specialist), a heart specialist, and others. The team acts as advisers to the person with diabetes.

Type 1 diabetes – the body no longer produces insulin (a hormone necessary for converting food into energy). In people with type 1 diabetes, the body's immune system attacks and destroys the insulin-producing cells in the pancreas (an integral part of the digestive system). The pancreas then produces little or no insulin. Only 5% of people with diabetes have type 1, and must take insulin (via injection or pump) to survive.

Type 2 diabetes – the most common type of diabetes, type 2 diabetes is a chronic illness that disrupts the way your body converts food into energy. For people with type 2 diabetes, the body usually still makes or uses insulin (a hormone necessary for converting food into energy), but doesn't produce enough insulin to overcome the insulin resistance of the tissues and, as a result, is not able to maintain a healthy blood glucose level.

When you eat, the body breaks down the sugars and starches in food into glucose (the basic fuel for your body's cells). Think of insulin as the key that unlocks the cells to receive glucose. When glucose builds up in the blood instead of going into cells (with the help of insulin), your body doesn't get the energy it needs to function, and you are at risk for health complications.

Type 2 diabetes can be managed through lifestyle choices—nutrition, exercise, and stress and sick day management—and may require medication (pills or eventually insulin).

II. THE POWER OF TED* TERMS

The Dreaded Drama Triangle (DDT): Victim, Persecutor, Rescuer—Based on Stephen Karpman's original Karpman Drama Triangle, the DDT involves three intertwined roles.

1. **Victim.** The central figure in the DDT, a Victim is one who feels powerless and has experienced some loss, thwarted desire or aspiration, and/or the psychic death of a dream. An important distinction is made between *victimization*, which is a situation in which one is victimized to some degree, and *Victimhood*, which is a self-identity and "poor me" life stance.

2. **Persecutor.** The Persecutor serves as the cause of the Victim's perceived powerlessness, reinforcing the Victim's "Poor Me" identity. The Persecutor may be a person, condition (such as a health condition), or a circumstance (a natural disaster, for example).

3. **Rescuer.** The Rescuer is any person or activity (such as an addiction) that serves to help a Victim relieve the "pain" of Victimhood. As an activity, the Rescuer helps the Victim "numb out." Despite having helpful intentions, the Rescuer as a person reinforces the Victim's "Poor Me" by adopting a "Poor You" attitude, which serves to increase the Victim's sense of powerlessness. This renders the Victim dependent upon the Rescuer for a sense of safety.

FISBE – This serves as the basis of the "mental model" that underpins the two Orientations. It is an acronym for the three elements of the model: where people put their Focus engages in them an emotional Inner State, which then drives their Behavior. The two primary mental models (Victim and Creator) are referred to as "Orientations" because what we focus on (i.e., *orient* on) has a great deal to do with what manifests in our experience.

Victim Orientation – It is in this Orientation that the DDT thrives. In this way of being, one's Focus is on the *problem* or *problems* that dominate one's life. When a problem occurs, it engages an inner state of *anxiety,* which in turn causes one to *react*. There are three basic forms of reacting: *fight, flight,* or *freeze*. The DDT is based on fear, avoidance (of feelings, loss, pain, reality), and/or aggressive reactivity.

Creator Orientation – The alternative to the Victim Orientation, this is the way of being in which TED* (*The Empowerment Dynamic) is cultivated. The FISBe here is much different. A Creator consciously focuses on a *vision* or *outcome* — that which one chooses to create in their life. As they focus on what they want to manifest, a Creator taps into an inner state of *passion,* which propels them to take a *Baby Step* (the Behavior in this Orientation). Each small movement is either an advancement toward the vision or a clarification of the final form of the desired outcome. A Creator still faces and solves problems, but she does so in the course of creating the outcomes, rather than merely reacting to problems.

AIR – This acronym highlights the three key differences between the Victim and the Creator Orientation. The first is where you place your *Attention* (on what's wanted instead of what's not wanted). The second is what you hold as your *Intention* (manifesting outcomes, not just ridding yourself of problems). The third is *Results* (satisfying and sustainable, not temporary and reactive). The acronym AIR also serves to reinforce the reality that a very different experience and environment (hence, "air") is generated by each of the two orientations.

TED* (*The Empowerment Dynamic): Creator, Challenger, Coach - As a result of moving from the Victim Orientation to the Creator Orientation, a whole new set of roles and relationship dynamics becomes possible. The Empowerment Dynamic is made up of the following three roles, each of which serves as an antidote to the toxic roles of the DDT.

1. **Creator.** This is the central role of TED* and is the antidote to the powerless Victim. A Creator cultivates their capacity to create outcomes by adopting a Creator Orientation and harnessing Dynamic Tension. A Creator greatly increases their ability to choose a response to life circumstances (even in the harshest of situations),

rather than merely reacting to them. Creators seek and form relationships with other Creators (Co-Creators), both to support and to be supported through the other two roles that make up TED*.

2. **Challenger.** Serving as an antidote to a Persecutor which provokes a reaction from a Victim – a Challenger is a catalyst for change, learning, and growth for a Creator. A Challenger may be conscious and constructive, especially when in relationship with another Creator. Some of the Challengers we meet in life are unconscious—a person, condition, or circumstance that comes into our experience uninvited. In either case, a Creator is able to embrace the experience of a Challenger as a call to action, learning, and growth.

3. **Coach.** The antidote to a Rescuer – who reinforces the powerlessness of a Victim – a Coach views others as being creative and resourceful. A Coach sees each person they relate to as a Creator in their own right, and seeks to support them in the process of creating outcomes. A Coach does this by asking questions that help clarify envisioned outcomes, current realities, and possible Baby Steps. A Coach dares a Creator to dream and discern the pathways for manifesting their visions.

Harnessing Dynamic Tension – Adapted from the work of Robert Fritz *(The Path of Least Resistance)*,

Dynamic Tension is a way of planning for and taking action in creating outcomes. One begins by identifying and describing the *vision/outcome* they desire to create. The next step is to carefully and completely assess *current reality* as it relates to the envisioned outcome. There are two aspects of the current situation to identify. The first aspects are those things that are happening or exist that *support* and are helpful in the creation of the outcome. The second aspects are the problems, obstacles, or things that are missing that *inhibit* one's capacity to create the vision. By focusing on both the outcome and the current reality, one engages the tension — a creative force — between what they want and where they are. A Creator resolves this tension by taking *Baby Steps* to move from current reality toward the desired outcome. Each small step brings learning—whether it results in a step "back," a step "forward," or a "quantum leap"— in the process of creating outcomes.

Making Shifts Happen – Making shifts happen from the Victim to the Creator Orientation and from the DDT roles to their antidotes in TED* is the pathway for transforming how we experience life and interact in relationships. The shift from Victim to Creator takes place by focusing on what one wants, rather than what they don't want; by moving from reacting to choosing outcomes and one's responses to life experiences; and by reconnecting to one's dreams and desires. Transforming one's relationship with Persecutors so that they become Challengers, calls forth learning and growth. To become a conscious Challenger in relationship with others requires clarity of intention, the ability to see the other as a Creator in his own right, and the wish to provoke and evoke growth and development. The shift from Rescuer to Coach invites one to see the other as creative and resourceful, and to support them in the creation process by asking questions and facilitating their own clarification of envisioned outcomes, the current realities they face, and possible Baby Steps for moving forward.

Resources and Support

The following is a short list of resources for diabetes and the primary behavioral and psychological influencers of the TED* frameworks. For a more complete and growing list of resources, go to www.powerofTED.com/diabetes/.

Type 2 Diabetes

Online diabetes resources, with a variety of information for newly diagnosed to experienced people with diabetes.

American Diabetes Association
www.diabetes.org
Information and resources (including a book store)

Daily Strength
http://www.dailystrength.org/c/Diabetes-type-2/support-group
Supportive and innovative online community

dLife
www.dlife.com
Empowers diabetes self-management

DiaTribe
http://www.diatribe.us/home.php
Research and product news for people with diabetes

MedlinePlus
http://www.nlm.nih.gov/medlineplus/diabetes.html
News from the National Library of Medicine and the National Institutes of Health

TuDiabetes
http://www.tudiabetes.org
Supportive and innovative online community

Diabetes Professionals

Diabetes Mine Design Challenge
http://www.diabetesmine.com/category/products/the-design-challenge
Creative ideas for diabetes products

American Diabetes Association | Professional
http://professional.diabetes.org
For all diabetes professionals, scientific information and education

American Association of Diabetes Educators (AADE) http://www.diabeteseducator.org/
Information and education for diabetes educators

National Diabetes Education Initiative
http://www.ndei.org/website/

Resource for professionals caring for type 2 diabetes patients

National Diabetes Information Clearinghouse
http://diabetes.niddk.nih.gov/

Free downloads and publications for patients

American Association of Clinical Endocrinologists
http://www.aace.com/

Behavioral/Psychological Links

Karpman Drama Triangle: http://www.karpman-dramatriangle.com/ Dr. Karpman's website has information on the drama triangle. Also good information on Wikipedia: http://en.wikipedia.org/wiki/Karpman_drama_triangle

The Leadership Circle: http://www.theleadership-circle.com/resources/position-papers All of the position papers posted here are excellent. "Mastering Leadership" has the most direct reference to the Orientations.

Robert Fritz: http://www.robertfritz.com/ The originator of Structural Tension, upon which Dynamic Tension is based. The books that most influenced TED* are *The Path of Least Resistance* and *Creating*.

ACKNOWLEDGMENTS

The creation of this book is truly a testament to collaboration.

It began with the persistence of Dr. Scott over several years in encouraging me to apply TED* to health empowerment, to which he passionately committed. His support in my becoming an "activated patient" and in taking responsibility for my own physical health has been deeply appreciated.

Roy M Carlisle, our now years-long editor, publishing consultant and advocate, immediately got the vision when he heard of the idea for the book, given of his own relationship with diabetes and his deep understanding of the challenges of living with this disease. (He is truly one of the most activated patients I have ever met!). Roy connected us with Carmen Renee Berry, herself an accomplished author, who brought her writing support and art of storytelling to the narrative.

Ann Deaton, PhD and Sandra Smith, PhD – both TED* Practitioners with a deep interest in health literacy and empowerment – served as early readers, as did Kate Deaton. Other readers included Bill Fears, MD; Mary McNeill, CDE; and Bill Marsh, along with additional readers in Roy's and Scott's networks. All provided invaluable feedback.

One of the "little miracles" that occurred in the process of this project was the finding of consultant Colleen Broughton in our own backyard. Her experience in marketing and communications – including serving as the worldwide community director on diabetes for a major pharmaceutical corporation – has been an enormous contribution.

My time and ability to focus on writing would not have been possible without the support of the TED* Team, especially Kathy Haskin and Debbie Hulbert. You are the greatest!

Last, and by any measure, most importantly, deep gratitude to Donna Zajonc, my wife, partner and director of coaching and practitioner services for The Power of TED*. This project would never have come to fruition without your leadership and learning the ropes of publishing. And your commitment to your own health – as well as steady support of my own – is an inspiration. You are truly the mother of TED* in all that we are doing.

To all – named and unnamed – thank you for your unique contribution to this collaboration. You serve as an example of co-creating that is at the heart of TED* (*The Empowerment Dynamic)!

And, finally, I want to acknowledge the millions of us who face the Challenger of diabetes and the healthcare professionals who support and guide us in taking responsibility for our health.

David Emerald

There are times in your life when you are inspired to action.

Reading *The Power of TED** by David Emerald revealed an empowering and effective way to confront the challenges of life. Appreciating the struggle of those with diabetes, it became a mission to make sure they had access to David's work in the context of the challenges they face twenty four hours every day.

Watching David confront his diagnosis of diabetes, struggle with the implications for his life, and then to overcome diabetes confirmed the value of his work and the need to share with others.

Humbled by his vision, insight, and courage, it has been a tremendous honor to work with him on the creation of this book.

To those of you with diabetes I acknowledge and appreciate the challenges you face. It takes a special person to pass up flavorful food or get out and exercise when fatigue, habits, and medical illnesses make doing the right thing for your body seemingly impossible for a "normal" person.

Thank you for the dedication and fortitude it takes to face the odds and to do the right thing for yourself.

Thank you for being "abnormal" and taking the time to read this book, to choose health and wellness, and to be an inspiration for those who see you live a vital life despite of the challenges faced.

To the doctors, nurses, and health care staff that see people with diabetes, thank you for your commitment. Providers like Bill Fears, who dedicates his life to improving the life of his patients, and Mary McNeil, who comes up with new innovative ways to educate and motivate people to maintain or improve their quality of life. They are never discouraged, always optimistic that every person deserves a great life and the opportunity to learn and grow to confront and overcome life's challenges.

To the American Diabetes Association and American Academy of Endocrinology for their commitment to keeping diabetes in the minds of those in government, business, and the community. Their dynamic tension and willingness to insure that diabetes is at the forefront of the national conversation and that no person with diabetes goes without the opportunity to receive the treatment they need to manage and overcome their disease.

To the American Association of Diabetes Educators for their "dedication to integrating self-management as a key outcome in the care of people with diabetes and related chronic conditions."

To the researchers who study and find ways for us to identify people at risk so that we can support change and move from treating those with the diabetes to helping identify and act during the 5 – 15 year window before they develop diabetes so that the legacy of blindness, amputations and kidney failure can be prevented.

I acknowledge the risk and commitment the founders and funders of companies like Tethys Bioscience who take tremendous risk to do the research and provide tools to make prediabetes easier to identify and to intervene while there is still time.

Finally to Susan, my wife, who supported me during the writing of this book. A labor of love, she proofed and provided feedback at the dinner table, on vacation and in the car far more than she might have chosen voluntarily. Her honesty and encouragement provided the focus and dedication needed to complete this manuscript.

Scott Conard, M.D.

DAVID EMERALD
and *THE POWER OF TED**
PRODUCTS and SERVICES

Customer designed programs for:
- Team building • Retreats • Coaching
- Leadership Development • Strategic Planning
- Employee Engagement • Work/life Balance
- Health Empowerment

Keynote Speaking
Association meetings • Business retreats
• Wellness programs

Books, CD's and Workbooks
Workshops and Seminars
TED* Practitioner Program
TED* for Coaches Webinars

For further information contact:
The Power of TED*
321 High School Rd. D3, #295,
Bainbridge Island, WA USA 98110
206.780.9900
email: demerald@powerofted.com
www.powerofted.com

SCOTT CONARD, M.D.
and GAME OF HEALTH
PRODUCTS and SERVICES

Services and Programs
GOH4Wellness, a subscription based wellness program delivered digitally with assessment, learning, and live coaching.
GOH4Health, a subscription based local health and wellness program available to patients without insurance.
GOH4Breakthroughs, a monthly health and wellness series taught in Dallas, TX.

Books
Weight Loss The Jabez Way • The Seven Healers • The Seven Numbers

Other
Executive concierge health program
• Keynote speaking
• Corporate healthcare consulting
• Hospital consulting

Contact Us
Game Of Health
923 Parkview Lane, Southlake, TX 76092
email: support@gameofhealth.com
GameOfHealth.com

ABOUT THE AUTHORS

David Emerald Womeldorff is a consultant, master facilitator, executive coach, speaker, and author. David's authentic style of presenting challenges individuals and groups to move beyond problem-oriented reactivity.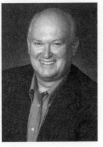

He is co-founder of the Bainbridge Leadership Center (Bainbridge Island, WA), along with his wife, Donna Zajonc. As director of the Center's Organizational Leadership and Self Leadership practice areas, David facilitates individuals, teams, and organizations in making conscious shifts toward leading and working from an outcome-focused orientation.

Writing under the pen name of David Emerald, he is the author of *The Power of TED* (*The Empowerment Dynamic*), a teaching story about Self Leadership, as well as the book's supplemental workbook, *A Personal Guide to Applying The Power of TED*. *The Power of TED* is also available as an ebook.

Scott E. Conard, MD, DABFM, FAAFP, is an author, speaker, and lectures internationally. He has more than twenty-five years of successful clinical practice, research, medical communications and leadership experience. Dr. Conard is dedicated to working with healthcare providers, corpo- 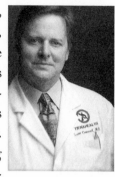 rations and individuals to add years to their life and life to their years by empowering them to take control of their health.

Currently he is the Chief Medical Officer of ACAP Health (www.acaphealth.com) and Holmes Murphy & Associates (www.holmesmurphy.com) where he works with corporations, the public sector, and healthcare providers to create systems of Accountable Care (AC) and Accountable Patients (AP) that ensure high value (= safety + quality/cost) for all employees.

Dr. Conard has been active on the Board of the North Texas Chapter of the American Diabetes Association (ADA). He is the 2012 President of the North Texas Chapter and on the 2012 ADA National Committee on Prevention. He is a diplomat of the American Board of Family Practice and a Fellow of the American Academy of Family Medicine. He is board certified in Bariatric (weight loss) Medicine, and in Behavioral Sleep Medicine and Diabetes Education (as a Certified Diabetic Educator). He has remained active in teaching as an Associate Clinical Professor at University of Texas Southwestern Medical School Department of Family Practice and Community Medicine.

Dr. Conard has hosted a weekly television talk show (Health Connection), a weekly radio show "All About Life Radio" and has appeared regularly on health related radio and television news programs.

Dr. Conard is a graduate of the University of South Florida Medical School, the Stegan Institute, and has studied business and management at the University of Dallas School of Business.